Activities & Assessment Manual

Fourth Edition

Jerome E. Kotecki
Ball State University
Muncie, Indiana

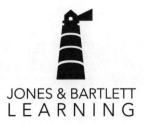

JONES & BARTLETT
LEARNING

World Headquarters
Jones & Bartlett Learning
5 Wall Street
Burlington, MA 01803
978-443-5000
info@jblearning.com
www.jblearning.com

Jones & Bartlett Learning books and products are available through most bookstores and online booksellers. To contact Jones & Bartlett Learning directly, call 800-832-0034, fax 978-443-8000, or visit our website, www.jblearning.com.

Substantial discounts on bulk quantities of Jones & Bartlett Learning publications are available to corporations, professional associations, and other qualified organizations. For details and specific discount information, contact the special sales department at Jones & Bartlett Learning via the above contact information or send an email to specialsales@jblearning.com.

Production Credits
Publisher: William Brottmiller
Acquisitions Editor: Megan R. Turner
Senior Editorial Assistant: Sean Coombs
Production Editor: Jessica Steele Newfell
Senior Marketing Manager: Jennifer Stiles
VP, Manufacturing and Inventory Control: Therese Connell
Composition: Cenveo® Publisher Services
Cover Design: Kristin E. Parker
Director of Photo Research and Permissions: Amy Wrynn
Cover Images: © Peter Hurley Studio/Chicago
Printing and Binding: Courier Companies
Cover Printing: Courier Companies

ISBN 978-1-4496-9345-9

6048
Printed in the United States of America
17 16 15 14 13   10 9 8 7 6 5 4 3 2 1

Contents

Chapter	Assignment	Page	Due Date	Complete

Preface

This manual provides a practical framework for you to individually apply the concepts outlined in *Physical Activity & Health: An Interactive Approach, Fourth Edition.* An important step in applying this knowledge is starting with a baseline assessment of your current health status, fitness status, and daily habits. To assist, I have put together more than 70 science-based health and fitness activities and assessments that examine your current status and measure what you are doing now. Completing each activity and assessment will help you identify the aspects of your personal behavior that with modification can improve your overall health.

Your instructor will provide directions indicating which activities and assessments are required assignments and the order and date(s) in which they are due. Each activity and assessment is self-explanatory. I encourage you to complete sections that are not required—now or in the future—on your own to fully recognize your areas of strength and your opportunities for improvement. By identifying areas needing improvement, you will be better able to set personal goals that allow for health enhancement.

To reach your personal goals, it helps to have a map to know where you are heading, the best way to get there, and the ways to travel without getting lost or running into detours. The "Ready, Set, Goals!" activity beginning on page 23 and the "Self-Contract" activity on page 33 provide such a map. These activities are tailored to the specific stages of readiness to change behavior. These activities chart a path that puts you in control of your behavior and allow you to decide what to do and how and when to do it.

Finally, I know that completing this manual will provide you with many opportunities for individual reflection as it relates to the management of your health. Self-reflecting on the way you are living will better allow your actions to come naturally into alignment with your sense of what is best for you to create health and happiness.

Name: _____ Course Number: _____

Section: _____ Date: _____

Healthstyle: A Self-Test

Directions: Answer the following questions regarding each dimension of health. Indicate how often you think the statements describe you using the scale below.

1 = Rarely, if ever
2 = Sometimes
3 = Most of the time
4 = Always

Physical Health

1. I accumulate at least 150 minutes (2 hours and 30 minutes) of moderate-intensity aerobic activity or 75 minutes (1 hour and 15 minutes) of vigorous-intensity aerobic activity every week or an equivalent mix of moderate- and vigorous-intensity aerobic activity. 1 2 3 4

2. I include muscle-strengthening activities on 2 or more days a week that work all major muscle groups (legs, hips, back, abdomen, chest, shoulders, and arms). 1 2 3 4

3. I maintain a healthy body weight, which includes evaluating my waist circumference periodically to ensure that fat is not accumulating around my waist. 1 2 3 4

4. I consume a variety of fruits and vegetables each day. In particular, I select from all five vegetable subgroups—dark green, orange, legumes, starchy vegetables, and other vegetables—several times a week. 1 2 3 4

5. I choose my dietary fats wisely by consuming less than 10 percent of my daily calories from saturated fatty acids and less than 300 milligrams per day of cholesterol and keep trans fatty acid consumption below 2 grams daily while eating more monounsaturated and polyunsaturated fats and oils. 1 2 3 4

6. I avoid smoking cigarettes. 1 2 3 4

7. If I choose to drink alcohol, I do so in moderation. 1 2 3 4

8. I have regular check-ups and age-appropriate health screenings completed by health care providers to identify potential health problems early. 1 2 3 4

9. I regularly take steps to avoid injuries (e.g., wearing a safety belt while riding in a car, wearing a helmet while riding a bike). 1 2 3 4

10. I get between 7–9 hours of sleep most nights. 1 2 3 4

1 = Rarely, if ever
2 = Sometimes
3 = Most of the time
4 = Always

Social Health

1. When I meet people, I feel good about the impression I make on them.   1 2 3 4

2. I am open, honest, and get along well with other people.   1 2 3 4

3. I participate in a wide variety of social activities and enjoy being with people who are different from me.   1 2 3 4

4. I try to be a "better person" and work on behaviors that have caused problems in my interactions with others.   1 2 3 4

5. I get along well with the members of my family.   1 2 3 4

6. I am a good listener.   1 2 3 4

7. I am open and accessible to a loving and responsible relationship.   1 2 3 4

8. I have someone I can talk to about my private feelings.   1 2 3 4

9. I consider the feelings of others and do not act in hurtful or selfish ways.   1 2 3 4

10. I consider how what I say might be perceived by others before I speak.   1 2 3 4

Emotional Health

1. I find it easy to laugh about things that happen in my life.   1 2 3 4

2. I avoid using alcohol as a means of helping me forget my problems.   1 2 3 4

3. I can express my feelings without feeling silly.   1 2 3 4

4. When I am angry, I try to let others know in nonconfrontational and and nonhurtful ways.   1 2 3 4

5. I am not a chronic worrier and do not tend to be suspicious of others.   1 2 3 4

6. I recognize when I am stressed and take steps to relax through exercise, quiet time, or other activities.   1 2 3 4

7. I feel good about myself and believe others like me for who I am.   1 2 3 4

8. When I am upset, I talk to others and actively try to work through my problems.   1 2 3 4

9. I am flexible and adapt or adjust to change in a positive way.   1 2 3 4

10. My friends regard me as a stable, emotionally well-adjusted person.   1 2 3 4

Environmental Health

1. I am concerned about environmental pollution and actively try to preserve and protect natural resources.   1 2 3 4

2. I report people who intentionally hurt the environment.   1 2 3 4

3. I recycle my garbage.   1 2 3 4

4. I reuse plastic and paper bags and tin foil.   1 2 3 4

5. I vote for pro-environment candidates in elections.   1 2 3 4

6. I write my elected leaders about environmental concerns.   1 2 3 4

7. I consider the amount of packing covering a product when I buy groceries.   1 2 3 4

8. I try to buy products that are recyclable.   1 2 3 4

9. I use both sides of the paper when taking class notes or doing assignments.   1 2 3 4

10. I try not to leave the faucet running too long when I brush my teeth, shave, or bathe.   1 2 3 4

Spiritual Health

1. I believe life is a precious gift that should be nurtured.   1 2 3 4

2. I take time to enjoy nature and the beauty around me.   1 2 3 4

3. I take time alone to think about what's important in life— who I am, what I value, where I fit in, and where I'm going.   1 2 3 4

4. I have faith in a greater power, be it a God-like force, nature, or the connectedness of all living things.   1 2 3 4

5. I engage in acts of caring and good will without expecting something in return.   1 2 3 4

6. I feel sorrow for those who are suffering and try to help them through difficult times.   1 2 3 4

7. I feel confident that I have touched the lives of others in a positive way.   1 2 3 4

8. I work for peace in my interpersonal relationships, in my community, and in the world at large.   1 2 3 4

9. I am content with who I am.   1 2 3 4

10. I go for the gusto and experience life to the fullest.   1 2 3 4

1 = Rarely, if ever
2 = Sometimes
3 = Most of the time
4 = Always

Intellectual Health

1. I think about consequences before I act.   1 2 3 4

2. I learn from my mistakes and try to act differently the next time.   1 2 3 4

3. I follow directions or recommended guidelines and act in ways likely to keep myself and others safe.   1 2 3 4

4. I consider the alternatives before making decisions.   1 2 3 4

5. I am alert and ready to respond to life's challenges in ways that reflect thought and sound judgment.   1 2 3 4

6. I do not let my emotions get the better of me when making decisions.   1 2 3 4

7. I actively learn all I can about products and services before making decisions.   1 2 3 4

8. I manage my time well rather than let time manage me.   1 2 3 4

9. My friends and family trust my judgment.   1 2 3 4

10. I think about my self-talk (the things I tell myself) and then examine the evidence to see if my perception and feelings are sound.   1 2 3 4

Occupational Health

1. I am happy with my career choice.   1 2 3 4

2. I look forward to working in my career area.   1 2 3 4

3. The job responsibilities/duties of my career choice are consistent with my values.   1 2 3 4

4. The payoffs/advantages in my career choice are consistent with my values.   1 2 3 4

5. I am happy with the balance between my work time and leisure time.   1 2 3 4

6. I am happy with the amount of control I have in my work.   1 2 3 4

7. My work gives me personal satisfaction and stimulation.   1 2 3 4

8. I am happy with the professional/personal growth provided by my job.   1 2 3 4

9. I feel my job allows me to make a difference in the world.   1 2 3 4

10. My job contributes positively to my overall well-being.   1 2 3 4

Personal Checklist

Now total your scores in each of the health dimensions and compare them to the ideal scores. Which areas do you need to work on?

	Ideal Score	Your Score
Physical health	40	_____
Social health	40	_____
Emotional health	40	_____
Environmental health	40	_____
Spiritual health	40	_____
Intellectual health	40	_____
Occupational health	40	_____

What Your Scores Mean

Scores of 35–40 points: Excellent. Your answers show that you are aware of the importance of this area to your health. More important, you are putting your knowledge to work for you by practicing good health habits. As long as you continue to do so, this area should not pose a serious health risk. It's likely that you are setting an example for your family and friends to follow. Although you reported a very high score on this part of the assessment, you may want to consider areas where your scores could be improved.

Scores of 30–34 points: Your health practices in this area are good, but there is room for improvement. Look again at the items you answered that scored one or two points. What changes could you make to improve your score? Even a small change in behavior can often help you achieve better health.

Scores of 20–29 points: Your health practices need improvement. Find information on how you could change these behaviors. Perhaps you need help deciding how to make the changes you desire. Assistance is available in this book, from your professor, and from resources on your campus.

Scores of 19 and lower: Your health practices need serious improvement and you may be taking unnecessary risks with your health. Perhaps you are not aware of the risks and what to do about them. In the textbook you will find the information you need to help improve your scores and your health.

Source: Adapted and modified from *Healthstyle: A Self-Test,* by USDHHS Publication Number (PHS) 8150155.

Name: _____ Course Number: _____

Section: _____ Date: _____

Family Health History

Being aware of your family's health history, especially which relatives had or have serious chronic diseases or inherited conditions, can help you and your physician assess your risk of such diseases or conditions. As a result of having this information, you can make choices concerning your lifestyle now that may reduce the likelihood of developing these health problems in the future.

To compile your personal health history and design a health history diagram, start with your own health and that of your brothers and sisters. Then indicate health conditions that affect your mother and father and their brothers and sisters. After completing health information for that generation, collect information about your grandparents' health. You may be aware of some family members' health problems, such as heart disease, obesity, drug addiction, or mental health conditions. In other instances, however, you will need to speak with your relatives to determine whether they have or had diseases or conditions such as prostate or breast cancer, diabetes, hypertension, liver disease, and so on. If you are adopted or cannot find information about individual family members, you may have to leave blanks.

A sample family health history diagram is shown in this assessment. Note that it has spaces for a person to fill in his or her personal health and the health of siblings, parents, aunts, uncles, and grandparents. Of course, your diagram will reflect your family's makeup. After developing your personal health history diagram, answer the following questions.

1. If a particular disease or condition occurs repeatedly in your family, it may be the result of inherited and/or lifestyle factors that are common within your family. Such repeated occurrences may indicate that your risk of developing the disease or condition is greater than average. Which serious health problems occur more than once in your family health history?

_____

_____

_____

2. Which diseases or conditions in your family history do you think are related to lifestyle practices, such as food choices, lack of regular physical activity, or smoking?

_____

_____

_____

3. Are you aware of actions you can take that may reduce your risk of developing the health problems that often affect or have affected members of your family? If so, list those actions.

_____

_____

_____

4. The course of many diseases and conditions is influenced by lifestyle factors. Your physician can help you determine such factors. Therefore, consider discussing your family health history with your physician. Your physician can also provide advice concerning steps you can take to reduce your risk of developing the health problems that affect or have affected members of your family.

_____

_____

_____

Family Health History Example

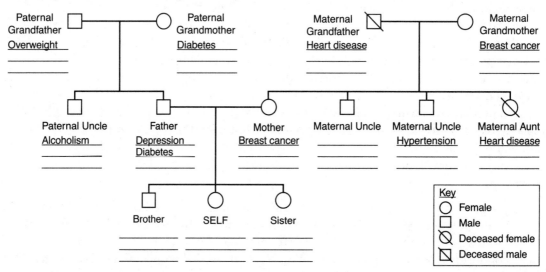

Family Health History

Name: ———————————————————————— Course Number: ————————————

Section: ———————————————————————— Date: ————————————

Defining Physical Activity and Health

You have had the opportunity to review several definitions regarding physical activity and health. Each person, however, defines physical activity and health according to his or her own values, goals, interests, and other factors that make that person unique. Respond to the following questions based on your personal definition of physical activity and health.

1. What is your personal definition of physical activity?

——————————————————————————————————————

——————————————————————————————————————

2. What is your personal definition of health?

——————————————————————————————————————

——————————————————————————————————————

3. Are there any similarities in these two definitions?

——————————————————————————————————————

——————————————————————————————————————

4. What aspects of your lifestyle reflect your definition of physical activity?

——————————————————————————————————————

——————————————————————————————————————

5. What aspects of your lifestyle reflect your definition of health?

——————————————————————————————————————

——————————————————————————————————————

6. What aspects of your lifestyle conflict with your definition of physical activity?

——————————————————————————————————————

——————————————————————————————————————

7. What aspects of your lifestyle conflict with your definition of health?

——————————————————————————————————————

——————————————————————————————————————

8. Describe three actions you plan to take that support your personal definition of physical activity and health.

_____

_____

_____

Source: Adapted from D. A. Birch and M. J. Cleary. (1996). *Managing Your Health: Assessment and Action.* Sudbury, MA: Jones & Bartlett.

Name: _____ Course Number: _____

Section: _____ Date: _____

Barriers to Being Active Quiz

Directions: Listed below are reasons that people give to describe why they do not get as much physical activity as they think they should. Please read each statement and indicate how likely you are to say each of the following statements:

3 = Very likely
2 = Somewhat likely
1 = Somewhat unlikely
0 = Very unlikely

How Likely Are You to Say . . .

1. My day is so busy now, I just don't think I can make the time to include physical activity in my regular schedule.   3 2 1 0

2. None of my family members or friends like to do anything active, so I don't have a chance to exercise.   3 2 1 0

3. I'm just too tired after work to get any exercise.   3 2 1 0

4. I've been thinking about getting more exercise, but I just can't seem to get started.   3 2 1 0

5. I'm getting older so exercise can be risky.   3 2 1 0

6. I don't get enough exercise because I have never learned the skills for any sport.   3 2 1 0

7. I don't have access to jogging trails, swimming pools, bike paths, etc.   3 2 1 0

8. Physical activity takes too much time away from other commitments—leisure time, work, family, etc.   3 2 1 0

9. I'm embarrassed about how I will look when I exercise with others.   3 2 1 0

10. I don't get enough sleep as it is. I just couldn't get up early or stay up late to get some exercise.   3 2 1 0

11. It's easier for me to find excuses not to exercise than to go out to do something.   3 2 1 0

12. I know of too many people who have hurt themselves by overdoing it with exercise.   3 2 1 0

13. I really can't see learning a new sport at my age. 　　　　3 2 1 0

14. It's just too expensive. You have to take a class or join a club or buy the right equipment. 　　　　3 2 1 0

15. My free times during the day are too short to include exercise. 　　　　3 2 1 0

16. My usual social activities with family or friends do not include physical activity. 　　　　3 2 1 0

17. I'm too tired during the week and I need the weekend to catch up on my rest. 　　　　3 2 1 0

18. I want to get more exercise, but I just can't seem to make myself stick to anything. 　　　　3 2 1 0

19. I'm afraid I might injure myself or have a heart attack. 　　　　3 2 1 0

20. I'm not good enough at any physical activity to make it fun. 　　　　3 2 1 0

21. If we had exercise facilities and showers at work, then I would be more likely to exercise. 　　　　3 2 1 0

Follow these instructions to score yourself:

- Enter the circled number in the spaces provided, putting together the number for statement 1 on line 1, statement 2 on line 2, and so on.

- Add the three scores on each line. Your barriers to physical activity fall into one or more of seven categories: lack of time, social influences, lack of energy, lack of willpower, fear of injury, lack of skill, and lack of resources. A score of 5 or higher in any category shows that this is an important barrier for you to overcome.

____ + ____ + ____ = _____
　1　　　8　　　15　　　　　　　Lack of time

____ + ____ + ____ = _____
　2　　　9　　　16　　　　　　　Social influence

____ + ____ + ____ = _____
　3　　　10　　　17　　　　　　Lack of energy

____ + ____ + ____ = _____
　4　　　11　　　18　　　　　　Lack of willpower

____ + ____ + ____ = _____
　5　　　12　　　19　　　　　　Fear of injury

____ + ____ + ____ = _____
　6　　　13　　　20　　　　　　Lack of skill

____ + ____ + ____ = _____
　7　　　14　　　21　　　　　　Lack of resources

Suggestions for Overcoming Physical Activity Barriers

Lack of Time

- Identify available time slots. Monitor your daily activities for one week. Identify at least three 30-minute time slots you could use for physical activity.

- Add physical activity to your daily routine. For example, walk or ride your bike to work or shopping, organize school activities around physical activity, walk the dog, exercise while you watch TV, park farther away from your destination, etc.

- Make time for physical activity. For example, walk, jog, or swim during your lunch hour, or take fitness breaks instead of coffee breaks.

- Select activities requiring minimal time, such as walking, jogging, or stairclimbing.

Social Influence

- Explain your interest in physical activity to friends and family. Ask them to support your efforts.

- Invite friends and family members to exercise with you. Plan social activities involving exercise.

- Develop new friendships with physically active people. Join a group, such as the YMCA or a hiking club.

Lack of Energy

- Schedule physical activity for times in the day or week when you feel energetic.

- Convince yourself that if you give it a chance, physical activity will increase your energy level; then try it.

Lack of Motivation

- Plan ahead. Make physical activity a regular part of your daily or weekly schedule and write it on your calendar.

- Invite a friend to exercise with you on a regular basis and write it on both your calendars.

- Join an exercise group or class.

Fear of Injury

- Learn how to warm up and cool down to prevent injury.

- Learn how to exercise appropriately considering your age, fitness level, skill level, and health status.

- Choose activities involving minimum risk.

Lack of Skill

- Select activities requiring no new skills, such as walking, climbing stairs, or jogging.

- Exercise with friends who are at the same skill level as you are.

- Find a friend who is willing to teach you some new skills.

- Take a class to develop new skills.

Lack of Resources

- Select activities that require minimal facilities or equipment, such as walking, jogging, jumping rope, or calisthenics.

- Identify inexpensive, convenient resources available in your community (community education programs, park and recreation programs, worksite programs, etc.).

Weather Conditions

- Develop a set of regular activities that are always available regardless of weather (indoor cycling, aerobic dance, indoor swimming, calisthenics, stair climbing, rope skipping, mall walking, dancing, gymnasium games, etc.).

- Look on outdoor activities that depend on weather conditions (cross-country skiing, outdoor swimming, outdoor tennis, etc.) as "bonuses"—extra activities possible when weather and circumstances permit.

Travel

- Put a jumprope in your suitcase and jump rope.

- Walk the halls and climb the stairs in hotels.

- Stay in places with swimming pools or exercise facilities.

- Join the YMCA or YWCA (ask about reciprocal membership agreements).

- Visit the local shopping mall and walk for half an hour or more.

- Bring an iPod and your favorite aerobic exercise mp3.

Family Obligations

- Trade babysitting time with a friend, neighbor, or family member who also has small children.

- Exercise with the kids—go for a walk together, play tag or other running games, get an aerobic dance or exercise DVD for kids (there are several on the market) and exercise together. You can spend time together and still get your exercise.

- Hire a babysitter and look at the cost as a worthwhile investment in your physical and mental health.

- Jump rope, do calisthenics, ride a stationary bicycle, or use other home gym equipment while the kids are busy playing or sleeping.

- Try to exercise when the kids are not around (e.g., during school hours or their nap time).
- Encourage exercise facilities to provide child care services.

Retirement Years

- Look upon your retirement as an opportunity to become more active instead of less. Spend more time gardening, walking the dog, and playing with your grandchildren. Children with short legs and grandparents with slower gaits are often great walking partners.
- Learn a new skill you've always been interested in, such as ballroom dancing, square dancing, or swimming.
- Now that you have the time, make regular physical activity a part of every day. Go for a walk every morning or every evening before dinner. Treat yourself to an exercycle and ride every day while reading a favorite book or magazine.

Source: Reproduced from *Promoting Physical Activity: A Guide for Community Action* (USDHHS, 1999).

Name: _____   Course Number: _____

Section: _____   Date: _____

Chapter 1: Critical Thinking Questions

The Physical Activity and Health Connection

1. Are you feeling lethargic and tired, like Destiny? Could it be because of lack of physical activity? If so, what physical activity are you currently doing? If not, what can you do to increase your physical activity? Develop a list of campus events or organizations that involve physical activity (e.g., hiking club, co-ed intramural volleyball, walking club, kick boxing). Investigate several of them to see which one best fits your needs and schedule. Begin adding this activity into your daily or weekly college routine.

2. Using the seven dimensions of health, identify two behaviors you do that would be an example of enhancing each dimension.

3. The morning newspaper headline is "Scientific studies indicate physical activity is important to health and quality of life." The article mentions studies from the *Prestigious International Health and Medicine Journal*. Later that day, you hear a local radio report suggesting that too much physical activity can lead to an instant heart attack, maybe even death. You are bombarded with health messages daily. What is your major source of health information? Television? If so, which shows in particular? Magazines? School? Friends? How carefully do you analyze health information? Do you believe most of what you read about health, or does it depend on the source?

_____

_____

_____

_____

_____

_____

_____

_____

_____

_____

_____

_____

Name: _____ Course Number: _____

Section: _____ Date: _____

Lifestyle Behavior Readiness Assessment

Directions: Read each of the following lifestyle behavior descriptions, and then select the statement from the list that best expresses your intention or current practice. Circle the letter(s) that signifies your level of readiness.

Codes for Stages of Readiness for Behavior Change	
PC = Precontemplation	Description of target behavior doesn't match my current behavior patterns, and I don't intend to change them to be more like it in the next 6 months.
C = Contemplation	Description of target behavior doesn't match my current behavior patterns, but I do intend to change them to be more like it in the next 6 months.
P = Preparation	Description of target behavior doesn't match my current behavior patterns, but I am motivated and confident that I can change them to be more like it in the next month.
A = Action	Description of target behavior is similar to my current behavior patterns, but I've been practicing this behavior for less than 6 months.
M = Maintenance	Description of target behavior is similar to my current behavior patterns, and I've been practicing this behavior for 6 months or longer.

Specific Health Behavior	Stage of Change				
1. Engage in 30 minutes of daily, preferably 10 minutes at a time, intermittent light- or moderate-intensity lifestyle physical activity at home, work, or by commute.	PC	C	P	A	M
2. Engage in moderate-intensity aerobic exercise for 30 minutes or more on at least 5 days a week for a total of 150 minutes or vigorous-intensity aerobic exercise for 20 minutes or more on at least 3 days a weeks for a total of 75 minutes or a combination of moderate- and vigorous-intensity exercise to achieve cardiorespiratory endurance benefits.	PC	C	P	A	M
3. Engage in muscle-strengthening exercises on 2 or more days a week that work all major muscle groups (legs, hips, back, abdomen, chest, shoulders, and arms).	PC	C	P	A	M
4. Engage in stretching exercises on 2 or more days a week that stretch all major muscle groups.	PC	C	P	A	M
5. Engage in functional fitness exercises that simultaneously use multiple muscles and joints to improve strength, balance, and agility.	PC	C	P	A	M
6. Limit daily sustained sitting time to lessen the effects of sedentarism on metabolic health.	PC	C	P	A	M
7. Take frequent breaks to interrupt and intersperse sustained sitting. Stand up occasionally and move about briefly every 30 minutes.	PC	C	P	A	M
8. Evaluate waist circumference periodically to ensure that fat is not accumulating around your waist.	PC	C	P	A	M
9. Evaluate body weight using the body mass index (BMI) periodically to ensure that you are at a healthy weight.	PC	C	P	A	M
10. Employ stress-management coping and relaxation techniques when feeling stressed or overwhelmed.	PC	C	P	A	M
11. Eat a variety of vegetables, especially dark-green and red and orange vegetables and beans and peas.	PC	C	P	A	M
12. Consume at least half of all grains as whole grains and/or increase whole-grain intake by replacing refined grains with whole grains.	PC	C	P	A	M
13. Consume fat-free or low-fat milk and milk products, such as milk, yogurt, cheese, or fortified soy beverages.	PC	C	P	A	M
14. Choose a variety of protein foods, which include seafood, lean meat and poultry, eggs, beans and peas, soy products, and unsalted nuts and seeds.	PC	C	P	A	M
15. Increase the amount and variety of seafood consumed by choosing seafood in place of some meat and poultry.	PC	C	P	A	M
16. Replace protein foods that are higher in solid fats with choices that are lower in solid fats and calories and/or are sources of oils. The fats in meat, poultry, and eggs are considered solid fats, while the fats in seafood, nuts, and seeds are considered oils. Meat and poultry should be consumed in lean forms to decrease intake of solid fats.	PC	C	P	A	M
17. Use oils to replace solid fats when possible.	PC	C	P	A	M

Specific Health Behavior	Stage of Change				
18. Choose foods that provide more potassium, dietary fiber, calcium, and vitamin D, which are nutrients of concern in American diets. These foods include vegetables, fruits, whole grains, and milk and milk products.	PC	C	P	A	M
19. Choose and prepare foods with little salt, and consume less than 2300 milligrams (mg) of sodium per day.	PC	C	P	A	M
20. Consume less than 10 percent of calories from saturated fatty acids by replacing them with monounsaturated and polyunsaturated fatty acids.	PC	C	P	A	M
21. Keep trans fatty acid consumption as low as possible by limiting foods that contain synthetic sources of trans fats, such as partially hydrogenated oils, and by limiting other solid fats.	PC	C	P	A	M
22. Limit the consumption of foods that contain refined grains, especially refined-grain foods that contain solid fats, added sugars, and sodium.	PC	C	P	A	M
23. If you consume alcohol, consume it in moderation—up to one drink per day for women and two drinks per day for men—and only if you are of legal drinking age.	PC	C	P	A	M
24. In communicating with your partner or close friends, send clear messages.	PC	C	P	A	M
25. In communicating with your partner or close friends, use effective listening techniques.	PC	C	P	A	M
26. If you and your partner have made a conscious decision to have sexual intercourse, use a condom every time.	PC	C	P	A	M
27. Choose not to smoke cigarettes.	PC	C	P	A	M
28. Choose not to smoke marijuana.	PC	C	P	A	M
29. Other:	PC	C	P	A	M
30. Other:	PC	C	P	A	M
31. Other:	PC	C	P	A	M

The responses in this assessment allow you to rate your level of readiness to change a number of health behaviors. It is common to be at various stages of change for different behaviors. Your goal is to begin thinking about one behavior that you would benefit from modifying. You will use the Ready Set Goals! worksheets from Activity 2.2. The Ready Set Goals! worksheets are tailored to specific stages of readiness to change behavior. Depending on your stage of readiness, your goals will be different.

Name: _____   Course Number: _____

Section: _____   Date: _____

Ready, Set, Goals!

This section contains four different goal-setting worksheets. The worksheets are tailored to specific stages of readiness to change behavior. Depending on your stage of readiness, your goals will be different.

Precontemplation or Contemplation

Your goal will be to begin thinking about the healthy lifestyle behavior you selected to work on. You will consider the ways you could benefit from practicing the behavior and think about how you could overcome any obstacles that are blocking you from achieving this goal. This worksheet provides a useful tool for weighing the costs and benefits associated with making a change. It also employs visualization as a technique for thinking about change. You are encouraged to eliminate negative "self-talk" ("I'm always so lazy") and replace it with positive "self-talk" ("I didn't work out last week, but I will today").

Preparation

Your goal will be to commit to the decision you made to change your behavior soon. You will do so by setting small, realistic goals and creating a plan to take action.

You will learn to write SMART goals—that is, goals that are *s*pecific, *m*easurable, *a*chievable, *r*elevant, and *t*rackable. For example, instead of setting a goal to "always eat breakfast," set a more realistic and achievable goal: "I will eat breakfast before Spanish class three mornings this week."

Action

Your goal will be to firmly establish the new behavior as a lifelong habit by anticipating problems and preparing to overcome failures, and by rewarding your successes to stay committed.

Maintenance

Your goal will be to stay focused and renew your commitment to the healthy behavior you selected to work on. You will consider new ways to achieve your goals for long-term health and identify ways to prevent the inevitable slip-ups from becoming full-fledged backslides.

These worksheets are adapted from the "wellStage" brochures developed by Health Enhancement Systems, Inc. (hesonline.com) and are used with permission. These tools are effective in changing not only eating and activity behaviors but also other health behaviors. You are welcome to use these behavior change worksheets in your future area of practice with credit given to the source.

PRECONTEMPLATION OR CONTEMPLATION

Assessment Area: _____

Current Behavior: _____

Target Behavior: _____

Your goal is to begin thinking about this healthy lifestyle behavior. You will consider the ways you could benefit from this behavior and think about how you could overcome any obstacles that are preventing you from practicing this behavior.

Step 1

Imagine that a friend or family member was told by his or her doctor to adopt this behavior. What advantages of this behavior would you highlight to motivate your friend or family member? (List at least three.)

_____

_____

_____

What are some things that might get in the way of this person's efforts to implement the target behavior? (List at least two.) What ideas do you have to help your friend or family member overcome these obstacles?

_____

_____

_____

What suggestions would you make to help this person get started? (What is one small, simple thing he or she could do every day?)

_____

_____

© 2014 Jones & Bartlett Learning

Step 2

Now consider your *own* costs and benefits for adopting this behavior. Fill in the grid on the next page. Which is *greater*, the left side—reasons to change—or the right side—reasons to stay the same?

_____ reasons to change _____ reasons to stay the same

What *one* benefit of the new behavior do you think will motivate you the most?

_____

_____

What *one* "cost" or barrier do you think will present the biggest obstacle for you?

_____

_____

Step 3

Being able to visualize performing the desired behavior is an important step in reshaping your beliefs, attitudes, and behaviors. Visualize yourself practicing the target behavior and all the associated preparation and implementation steps and imagine the subsequent feelings of health and confidence. Write down three distinct visual images of different aspects of practicing this behavior. (Examples include shopping, food preparation, and eating behaviors.) Use positive phrases of self-talk.

_____

_____

_____

Step 4

Start to recognize successes you achieve in practicing this behavior, no matter how small. Look over the records you kept. When were you successful in following the desired behavior even a little? Why do you think you were successful?

_____

_____

_____

Were there certain times of day, or situations, that prevented success? If so, what were they, and how might you prepare for these times so you can be more successful?

_____

_____

_____

Lifestyle Behavior Change: Perceived Costs and Benefits

Perceived Cost of Continuing Current Lifestyle Behavior *Why should I change?* *How is my current behavior hurting me?*	**Perceived Benefit of Continuing Current Lifestyle Behavior** *What do I give up if I change?*
Perceived Benefit of Adopting New Healthful Lifestyle Behavior *How will this new behavior help me?*	**Perceived Cost of Adopting New Healthful Lifestyle Behavior** *How much will this change "cost" or hurt?*

Ready, Set, Goals!

Step 5

Increasing your knowledge of the advantages of practicing this behavior and the disadvantages of failing to do so can help motivate you for change. What one thing can you learn more about?

_____

_____

Step 6

Other people can help or hinder the behavior change process. Identify at least one person who can support your efforts, and list one or more things he or she can do to provide support.

_____

_____

PREPARATION

Assessment Area: _____

Current Behavior: _____

Target Behavior: _____

Your goal is to commit to the decision you have made to change your behavior *soon*. You will do so by setting small, realistic goals and creating a plan to take action.

Step 1

How do you expect to benefit from adopting this behavior?

_____

_____

Which of these reasons is *most* important to you, and why?

_____

_____

Step 2

What changes will you need to make to achieve the target behavior? In other words, what will you need to do differently to succeed?

_____

_____

Step 3

Set goals to help you practice the target behavior. **SMART** goals have all of the following characteristics:

S (Specific)	Write down precisely what you want to achieve. Don't be vague.
M (Measurable)	Write down amounts, times, days, and any other measurable factors.
A (Achievable)	Your goal should be realistic—something that challenges you to stretch but is not impossible to achieve. Avoid the words *always* and *never*.
R (Relevant)	Your goal should be important to *you,* rather than simply done as an assignment for class.
T (Trackable)	Recording your progress helps you see what you've achieved and is one of the things that results in long-term success.

Write one or two SMART goals that will help you achieve the target behavior:

1. _____

2. _____

Step 4

Commit to take action. Set a start date. Pick a date at least 5 days before this part is due so that you can try out your goals and record the results of your efforts.

Start date: _____

Tell someone what you plan to do. Being accountable to others motivates you and also offers you the support and encouragement of others.

Who did you tell? _____

Signature: _____

Step 5

Track your progress. For 3 days after your start date, keep track of the results of trying to meet your SMART goal(s) on the following chart:

SMART Goals	Dates	Results

Step 6

Evaluate your progress and continue or modify your plan:

_____

_____

_____

_____

ACTION

Assessment Area: _____

Current Behavior: _____

Target Behavior: _____

Your goal is to firmly establish this behavior as a lifelong habit by anticipating problems and preparing to overcome failures, and by rewarding your successes to stay committed.

Step 1

In what ways have you benefited from adopting this behavior?

_____

_____

What motivates you the most to continue practicing this behavior, and why?

_____

_____

Step 2

What are some of the obstacles that you have encountered that make it difficult to consistently practice this behavior? (Common obstacles include stress, lack of time, travel, and boredom.) List each obstacle you encounter (or anticipate encountering), and identify one or more potential solutions to keep this obstacle from getting in your way of achieving your goal.

Obstacles	Solutions

Step 3

Set goals to help you continue to practice the target behavior. **SMART** goals have all of the following characteristics:

S (Specific)	Write down precisely what you want to achieve. Don't be vague.
M (Measurable)	Write down amounts, times, days, and any other measurable factors.
A (Achievable)	Your goal should be realistic—something that challenges you to stretch but is not impossible to achieve. Avoid the words *always* and *never*.
R (Relevant)	Your goal should be important to *you*, rather than simply done as an assignment for class.
T (Trackable)	Recording your progress helps you see what you've achieved and is one of the things that results in long-term success.

Write one or two SMART goals that will help you consistently achieve the target behavior:

1. _____

2. _____

Step 4

Reward your progress. Permanently changing lifestyle behaviors takes patience and consistent positive reinforcement. List several rewards you could give yourself for meeting your goals:

Select a reward for meeting your goal(s) for 3 days: _____

Step 5

Record your progress toward earning your reward. For 3 days, keep track of the results of trying to meet your SMART goal(s) on the following chart:

SMART Goals	Dates	Results

MAINTENANCE

Assessment Area: _____

Current Behavior: _____

Target Behavior: _____

Your goal is to stay focused and renew your commitment to this behavior. You will consider new ways to achieve your goals for long-term health, and identify ways to prevent the inevitable slip-ups from becoming full-fledged backslides.

Step 1

What benefits of practicing this behavior are most important to you, and why?

_____

_____

Step 2

How easy is this behavior to maintain? Is it truly a habit or do you need to expend some effort to do it?

_____

_____

Sometimes you might get off track briefly (but, hopefully, not permanently) and need to recommit yourself to a particular practice. How frequently do you *not* practice this particular behavior and why?

_____

_____

To prepare for these times, list several situations that might cause you to discontinue this behavior more often than once in a while. For each challenging situation, list one or more ideas to stay, or get back, on track.

Challenges	Solutions

Step 3

Try a new approach to achieving your goal (try a new food, a new recipe, a new activity, a change in routine). List at least two new things you could try:

1. _____

2. _____

Step 4

Record when you tried these new approaches and how it went:

New Approaches	Dates	Results

Step 5

If appropriate, consider writing a more challenging goal to achieve. Write your new goal:

_____

_____

_____

Source: Reproduced from B. Mayfield. (2006). *Personal Nutrition Profile,* 2nd ed. Sudbury, MA: Jones & Bartlett, 109–118.

Ready, Set, Goals!

Name: _____ Course Number: _____

Section: _____ Date: _____

Self-Contract

When you commit in writing what you want to accomplish, you increase the likelihood that you will act accordingly within a certain period of time. Eliciting this type of personal commitment has been shown to be one of the most important aspects of health behavior change, especially when you share this self-contract with others close to you.

Start date: _____ Finish date: _____

Goal: _____

Motivation (benefits): _____

Identify your current stage of change: _____

Match your current stage of change and other stages you anticipate progressing through with the appropriate processes of change:

_____   _____

_____   _____

What specific techniques will you use for each of the processes identified above?	
Processes	Specific Techniques
Stage of change on the finish date:	

Mini goals   Date   Reward

_____   _____   _____

_____   _____   _____

_____   _____   _____

I, _____, agree to work toward a healthier lifestyle and in doing so shall comply with the terms and dates of this contract.

Signature: _____ Date: _____

Witness: _____ Date: _____

Name: _____ Course Number: _____

Section: _____ Date: _____

Chapter 2: Critical Thinking Questions

Understanding and Enhancing Health Behaviors

1. Often, like Kevin, you might not be ready to make a health behavior change, especially if you think your effort will be greater than the benefit of the behavior. List 10 reasons people begin a physical activity program (benefits) and 10 reasons people do not begin a physical activity program (barriers). Put an *L* next to the benefits that are long term and a *B* next to those that are short term. Turning to the barriers, indicate which you have control over and which you do not. Do the barriers seem to outweigh the benefits? This time focus on short-term benefits and on barriers over which you have control. Does this change the picture?

2. As a friend, housemate, fraternity brother, or sorority sister, what role(s) can you play in supporting someone who is beginning a physical activity program? In analyzing your role, be aware of things you might do that would deter your friend from beginning or maintaining a physical activity program. Avoid those behaviors.

_____

_____

_____

_____

_____

_____

_____

_____

_____

_____

_____

_____

_____

_____

Critical Thinking Questions

© 2014 Jones & Bartlett Learning

Name: _____ Course Number: _____

Section: _____ Date: _____

PAR-Q and You: A Questionnaire for People Aged 15 to 69

Regular physical activity is fun and healthy, and more people are starting to become more active every day. Being more active is safe for most people. However, some people should check with their doctor before they start becoming much more physically active.

If you are planning to become much more physically active, start by answering the following seven questions.

If you are between the ages of 15 and 69, the PAR-Q will tell you if you should check with your doctor before you start. If you are older than 69 years of age, and you are not used to being very active, check with your doctor. Common sense is your best guide when you answer these questions. Please read the questions carefully and answer each one honestly: Check *yes* or *no*.

Yes   No

_____ _____ **1.** Has your doctor ever said that you have a heart condition *and* that you should only do physical activity recommended by a doctor?

_____ _____ **2.** Do you feel pain in your chest when you do physical activity?

_____ _____ **3.** In the past month, have you had chest pain when you were not doing physical activity?

_____ _____ **4.** Do you lose your balance because of dizziness or do you ever lose consciousness?

_____ _____ **5.** Do you have a bone or joint problem (e.g., back, knee, hip) that could be made worse by a change in your physical activity?

_____ _____ **6.** Is your doctor currently prescribing drugs (e.g., water pills) for your blood pressure or heart condition?

_____ _____ **7.** Do you know of *any other reason* why you should not do physical activity?

If You Answered YES to One or More Questions

Talk with your doctor by phone or in person *before* you start becoming much more physically active or *before* you have a fitness appraisal. Tell your doctor about the PAR-Q and which questions you answered YES.

- You may be able to do any activity you want—as long as you start slowly and build up gradually. Or, you may need to restrict your activities to those that are safe for you. Talk with your doctor about the kinds of activities in which you wish to participate and follow the doctor's advice.

- Find out which community programs are safe and helpful for you.

Delay Becoming Much More Active

- If you are not feeling well because of a temporary illness such as a cold or a fever—wait until you feel better; or

- If you are or may be pregnant—talk to your doctor before you start becoming more active.

If You Answered NO to All Questions

If you answered NO honestly to *all* PAR-Q questions, you can be reasonably sure that you can:

- Start becoming much more physically active—begin slowly and build up gradually. This is the safest and easiest way to go.

- Take part in a fitness appraisal—this is an excellent way to determine your basic fitness so that you can plan the best way for you to live actively. It is also highly recommended that you have your blood pressure evaluated. If your reading is over 144/94 mm Hg, talk with your doctor before you start becoming much more physically active.

> **Please Note:** If your health changes so that you then answer YES to any of the preceding questions, tell your fitness or health professional. Ask whether you should change your physical activity plan.

Informed Use of the PAR-Q: The Canadian Society for Exercise Physiology, Health Canada, and their agents assume no liability for persons who undertake physical activity, and, if in doubt after completing this questionnaire, consult your doctor prior to physical activity.

> You are encouraged to copy the PAR-Q, but only if you use the entire form.

Note: If the PAR-Q is being given to a person before he or she participates in a physical activity program or a fitness appraisal, this section may be used for legal or administrative purposes.

PAR-Q and You: A Questionnaire for People Aged 15 to 69

I have read, understood, and completed this questionnaire. Any questions I had were answered to my full satisfaction.

Name: _____

Signature: _____ Date: _____

Signature of Parent: _____ Witness: _____
or Guardian (for participants under the age of majority)

Source: Reproduced from *Physical Activity Readiness Questionnaire (PAR-Q).* © 2002. Used with permission from the Canadian Society for Exercise Physiology. Online: http://www.csep.ca/forms.asp.

Name: _____   Course Number: _____

Section: _____   Date: _____

Medical History Questionnaire

Directions: This questionnaire is designed to provide your exercise and physical activity professional with information necessary to assist you in the development of a physical activity program. It is not designed as a medical screening device. It is strongly suggested that you check with your physician before making any significant changes in your physical activity status.

Name: _____

         LAST NAME   FIRST NAME   MI

Address: _____

_____

_____

Phone number: _____

         HOME   WORK   EXT

Sex: _____ Date of birth: _____ Height: _____ Weight: _____

Name of physician: _____

Physician's address: _____

_____

Physician's phone number: _____

Person to contact in case of emergency: _____

Contact's address: _____

_____

Contact's phone number: _____

Any medications, foods, or other substances to which you are allergic:

_____

_____

When was the last time you had a physical examination? _____

Please list any chronic or serious illnesses you have as diagnosed by your physician.

_____

_____

_____

_____

Please list any operations you have had.

_____

_____

_____

Please list any hospitalizations lasting more than 1 day that you have had (other than normal pregnancies for women).

_____

_____

_____

Please list any prescription medications you are currently taking.

_____

_____

_____

Please list any over-the-counter medications you are currently taking.

_____

_____

_____

Have you experienced any of the following symptoms in the past
12 months?

	Yes	No
Fainting, light-headedness, or blackouts	_____	_____
Dyspnea or trouble breathing	_____	_____
Unusual difficulty sleeping	_____	_____
Blurred vision	_____	_____
Severe headaches or migraines	_____	_____
Chronic coughing	_____	_____
Slurring or loss of speech	_____	_____
Unusual nervousness or anxiety	_____	_____
Unusual heartbeats, skipped beats, or palpitations	_____	_____
Sudden tingling, numbness, or loss of sensation	_____	_____
Cold feet and hands in warm weather	_____	_____
Swelling of the feet and/or ankles	_____	_____
Pains or cramps in the legs	_____	_____
Pain or discomfort in the chest	_____	_____
Pressure or heaviness in the chest	_____	_____

Has a physician ever told you that you have any of the following
conditions?

	Yes	No
High blood pressure	_____	_____
Diabetes	_____	_____
High cholesterol	_____	_____
High triglycerides	_____	_____
Heart attack	_____	_____
Stroke	_____	_____
Arteriosclerosis	_____	_____
Heart murmur	_____	_____
Angina	_____	_____
Rheumatic fever	_____	_____
Aneurysm	_____	_____
Cancer	_____	_____
Abnormal ECG	_____	_____
Emphysema	_____	_____
Epilepsy	_____	_____
Arthritis	_____	_____

Has any member of your immediate family (parents, brothers, sisters, children, grandparents) ever been treated for, or died from, any of the following conditions?

	Yes	No
Diabetes	___	___
Heart disease	___	___
Stroke	___	___
High blood pressure	___	___
Do you smoke tobacco products?	___	___
If yes, how many per day? ___		

Name: _____   Course Number: _____

Section: _____   Date: _____

President's Challenge Adult Fitness Test

The President's Challenge is the premier program of the President's Council on Fitness, Sports, and Nutrition. One of the council's programs is the President's Challenge Adult Fitness Test, which measures an adult's aerobic fitness, muscular strength, flexibility, and body composition.

To assess your aerobic fitness you will either participate in a 1-mile walk or 1.5-mile run. To assess your muscular strength and endurance you will see how many pushups and sit-ups you can complete in one minute. To assess flexibility, your reach in the sit-and-reach test will be measured. To assess body composition, your body mass index (BMI) and waist circumference will be measured. Specifics on how to do each test properly for an accurate measure can be found at www.adultfitnesstest.org.

Once you have completed the tests, record your results on the form that follows. Enter your data online to receive an evaluation of your fitness level. After your scores have been calculated, record your results and percentiles in the table provided.

Fitness Component	Test Event	Your Results	Your Score
Aerobic Fitness	1-mile walk		
	Heart rate		
	VO_2 max		
Muscular Strength	Half sit-ups		
	Pushups		
Flexibility	Sit-and-reach		
Overall Score (based on percentile average)			
Body Composition	BMI		
	Waist circumference		

Interpret your scores: _____

_____

_____

When evaluating your performance, you should look at your results on each of the tests and consider how the individual tests contribute to your overall fitness. Your percentile scores are based on normative data, which represent the average achievement of people in your age group performing the test. For example, if your score is in the 75th percentile that means that 75 percent of the scores among people your age fall below your score. In general, the better you score on each test, the more fit you are. On the other hand, it is not necessary to score at the very highest level on all of the tests to be at reduced risk for a number of diseases. Scoring poorly on one test may help you identify specific fitness activities you need to do to improve your fitness score on that test. However, this does not mean you should ignore the fitness activities associated with the tests on which you performed well. Your goal should be to score well on as many of the fitness test items as possible, maintain your fitness level in those you did well, and improve the rest.

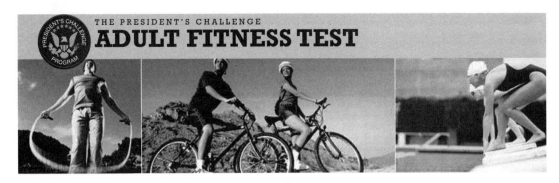

THE PRESIDENT'S CHALLENGE
ADULT FITNESS TEST

Get Your Adult Fitness Test Score!

As you complete each of the testing events, enter your data into the fields below. When all testing events are completed, transfer the data to the online data entry form and submit your data.

Please complete the form below. Mandatory fields are marked *

PERSONAL INFORMATION

State* ☐

Gender * ☐ Male   ☐ Female

Age * ☐ yrs

AEROBIC FITNESS

Must enter either a 1-mile walk time and heart rate or enter a 1.5-mile run time.

Mile Walk Time ☐ minutes ☐ seconds

Heart Rate (after walk) ☐ beats per minute

Weight ☐ lbs required for result calculation

OR

1.5-Mile Run Time ☐ minutes ☐ seconds

MUSCULAR STRENGTH

Half Sit-Ups ☐ (in one minute)

Push-Ups ☐

FLEXIBILITY

Sit and Reach ☐ inches

BODY COMPOSITION

BMI/BODY MASS INDEX

Enter height in feet AND inches.

Height ☐ feet ☐ inches

Weight ☐ lbs

Waist Measurement ☐ inches

Source: Reproduced from The President's Council on Fitness, Sports, & Nutrition. U.S. Department of Health and Human Services. The President's Challenge Adult Fitness Test. www.adultfitnesstest.org. Reprinted with permission.

Chapter 3: Critical Thinking Questions

Principles of Physical Fitness Development

1. Explain the differences between health-related fitness and skill-related fitness.

2. There are several scientific fitness principles (overload, progression, specificity, reversibility, recovery, individual differences) that you must adhere to in order to develop an effective physical activity program. Select three different principles and explain them.

3. You can use the FITT formula to help you determine how much exercise is enough for you to build fitness safely and effectively. What does FITT stand for?

———

———

———

———

———

———

———

———

———

———

———

———

———

———

———

———

———

———

———

Cardiorespiratory Exercise Readiness and Goal Setting

Directions: Indicate your stage of change in Step 1 and complete Steps 2, 3, 4, or 5, depending on which ones apply to your stage of change.

Step 1: Your Stage of Behavior Change

Please indicate which of the following statements best describes your readiness to follow the American College of Sports Medicine's recommendation for cardiorespiratory endurance exercise of engaging in "moderate-intensity aerobic exercise for 30 minutes or more on at least 5 days a week for a total of 150 minutes or vigorous-intensity aerobic exercise for 20 minutes or more on at least 3 days a weeks for a total of 75 minutes or a combination of moderate- and vigorous-intensity exercise to achieve cardiorespiratory benefits."

_____ Description of the cardiorespiratory exercise recommendation doesn't match my current behavior patterns, and I don't intend to change them to be like it in the next 6 months. (Precontemplation)

_____ Description of the cardiorespiratory exercise recommendation doesn't match my current behavior patterns, but I do intend to change them to be like it in the next 6 months. (Contemplation)

_____ Description of the cardiorespiratory exercise recommendation doesn't match my current behavior patterns, but I am motivated and confident that I can change them to be like it in the next month. (Preparation)

_____ Description of the cardiorespiratory exercise recommendation is similar to my current behavior patterns, but I've been practicing this behavior for less than 6 months. (Action)

_____ Description of the cardiorespiratory exercise recommendation is similar to my current behavior patterns, and I've been practicing this behavior for 6 months or longer. (Maintenance)

Step 2: Precontemplation or Contemplation

Your goal is to begin thinking about this exercise recommendation. You will consider the ways you could benefit from this behavior and think about how you could overcome any obstacles that are preventing you from practicing this behavior.

Imagine that a friend or family member was told by his or her health care provider to adopt this exercise recommendation. What advantages of this exercise recommendation would you highlight to motivate your friend or family member? (List at least three.)

_____

_____

What are some things that might get in the way of this person's efforts to implement this exercise recommendation? (List at least two.) What ideas do you have to help your friend or family member overcome these obstacles?

_____

_____

Now consider your own costs and benefits for adopting this exercise recommendation.

Reasons to Change

1. _____
2. _____
3. _____
4. _____
5. _____

Reasons to Stay the Same

1. _____
2. _____
3. _____
4. _____
5. _____

What one benefit of this exercise recommendation do you think will motivate you the most?

_____

_____

What one "cost" or barrier do you think will present the biggest obstacle for you?

_____

_____

Other people can help or hinder the behavior change process. Identify at least one person who can support your efforts, and list one or more things he or she can do to provide support.

_____

_____

Cardiorespiratory Exercise Readiness and Goal Setting

Step 3: Preparation

Your goal is to commit to this exercise recommendation soon. You will do so by setting small, realistic goals and creating a plan to take action.
What changes will you need to make to achieve this exercise recommendation? In other words, what will you need to do differently to succeed?

_____

_____

Write one or two SMART goals that will help you achieve this exercise recommendation:

1. _____

2. _____

Commit to take action. Set a start date: _____

Tell someone what you plan to do. Being accountable to others motivates you and also offers you support and encouragement.

Who did you tell? _____

Signature: _____

Step 4: Action

Your goal is to firmly establish this behavior as a lifelong habit by anticipating problems and preparing to overcome failures, and by rewarding your success to stay committed.

Track your progress. For 7 days after your start date, keep track of the results of trying to meet your SMART goal(s) on the following chart:

Smart Goals	Dates	Results

Evaluate your progress and continue or modify your plan:

_____

_____

In what ways have you benefited from adopting this behavior?

_____

_____

What motivates you the most to continue practicing this behavior and why?

_____

_____

Reward your progress. Permanently changing lifestyle behaviors takes patience and consistent positive reinforcement. List several rewards you could give yourself for meeting your goals:

_____

_____

Select a reward for meeting your goal(s) for 7 days: _____

Select a reward for meeting your goal(s) for 1 month: _____

Step 5: Maintenance

Your goal is to stay focused and renew your commitment to this behavior. You will consider new ways to achieve your goals for long-term health and identify ways to prevent the inevitable slip-ups from becoming full-fledged backslides.

What benefits of practicing this exercise recommendation are most important to you, and why?

_____

_____

How easy is this exercise recommendation to maintain? Is it truly a habit or do you need to expend some effort to do it?

_____

_____

Sometimes you might get off track briefly (but hopefully not permanently) and need to recommit yourself to this exercise recommendation. How frequently do you not meet this exercise recommendation and why?

_____

_____

Name: _____ Course Number: _____

Section: _____ Date: _____

Calculating Your Target Heart Rate Range Using the Heart Rate Reserve Method for Cardiorespiratory Endurance Activities

Step 1:

Calculate your estimated maximal heart rate (MHR) according to the following formula:

MHR = 207 − (.7 × age)*

Example for a 22-year-old: MHR = 207 − (.7 × 22) = 191.6 beats per minute (bpm)

Your MHR = 207 − (.7 × _____) = _____ bpm

* Research indicates that the traditional formula of (220 − age) overpredicts MHR in people 40 years and younger and underpredicts MHR in older individuals.

Step 2:

Determine your resting heart rate (RHR). Using either your carotid or radial artery, take your pulse as soon as you wake up and before you get out of bed in the morning. Take your pulse for 1 full minute, counting each heartbeat to find your bpm. For a more accurate measurement, take your pulse for three mornings and take the average by adding the three readings together and dividing that number by three. For example, Monday = 64, Tuesday = 66, Wednesday = 65.

RHR = 64 + 66 + 65 = 195/3 = 65 bpm

RHR = _____ + _____ + _____ = _____ /3 = _____ bpm

Finding Your Carotid Pulse

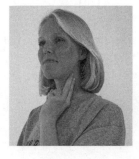

1. Turn your head to one side.

2. Feel the point at your neck where the large muscle and tendon stick out when your head is turned.

3. Slide the fleshy part of your index, middle, and ring fingers along this tendon until you are on a level equal to your Adam's apple.

4. Feel for the pulse. Readjust your fingers if necessary. Don't press too hard because this might alter your pulse.

5. Count the number of beats you feel for 60 seconds. This number represents your heart rate in bpm. If you are rushed for time, you can count the number of pulses you feel in 15 seconds and multiply by 4. Remember, however, that it is more accurate to take a full 60-second count if possible.

Finding Your Radial Pulse

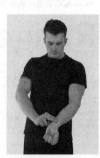

1. Hold your forearm out in front of you with your palm facing up.

2. Extend your wrist (move the back of your hand toward the back of your forearm).

3. At the top portion of your forearm (nearest your thumb) you should see, or at least be able to feel, a tendon just below your wristbone. This is the radial tendon. Your radial pulse can be found just about your radial tendon near the wrist.

4. Slide the fleshy part (fingertips) of your index, middle, and ring fingers (not your thumb) along this tendon until they are 1 inch from your wrist.

5. Use your fingertips, not your thumb, to find your pulse at the radial artery (at your wrist below your thumb).

6. Count the number of beats you feel for 60 seconds. This number represents your heart rate in bpm. If you are rushed for time, you can count the number of pulses you feel in 15 seconds and multiply by 4. Remember, however, that it is more accurate to take a full 60-second count if possible.

Note: If you need to use the bathroom when you wake up, do so, and then lie back down for a few minutes. Then take your heart rate, as a full bladder can increase your heart rate. RHR is also useful information to monitor your training and health. With improvement in your fitness level you should see your RHR decrease. Likewise a RHR 10 percent above your normal level usually indicates you are overtraining and/or sick and additional rest is required.

Step 3:

Calculate your heart rate reserve according to the following formula:

Heart rate reserve (HRR) = MHR – RHR.

HRR = _____ – _____ = _____ bpm

For example, a 22-year-old with a resting heart rate of 65 bpm would have a HRR of 126.6 (191.6 – 65 = 126.6).

Step 4:

Calculate your target heart using the following formulas based on the three intensity classifications provided:

Intensity	Formula	Calculated Heart Rates
Light	Lower limit = HRR × .30 + RHR	Lower = _____ bpm
	Upper limit = HRR × .39 + RHR	Upper = _____ bpm
Moderate	Lower limit = HRR × .40 + RHR	Lower = _____ bpm
	Upper limit = HRR × .59 + RHR	Upper = _____ bpm
Vigorous	Lower limit = HRR × .60 + RHR	Lower = _____ bpm
	Upper limit = HRR × .89 + RHR	Upper = _____ bpm

For example, a 22-year-old with a HRR of 126.6 bpm and a resting heart rate of 65 bpm interested in exercising at a moderate intensity range would have a lower limit of 115.6 bpm (126.6 × .40 + 65 = 115.6) and an upper limit of 139.7 bpm (126.6 × .59 + 65 = 139.7).

Note: Target Heart Rate Training is a systematic method of measuring your cardiorespiratory intensity. The method provides estimates of intensity. If you feel yourself becoming exceedingly exhausted, then you are working out too hard and should ease off. Individuals just starting an exercise program or with low cardiorespiratory fitness levels are encouraged to employ a light intensity. Individuals with fair or average cardiorespiratory fitness levels are encouraged to employ a moderate intensity. Active individuals with good or excellent cardiorespiratory fitness levels are encouraged to employ a vigorous intensity.

4.3

Name: _____ Course Number: _____

Section: _____ Date: _____

Cardiorespiratory Endurance Training Log

Directions: Track and record your cardiorespiratory endurance progress by date, activity, intensity, and duration.

Date	Activity	Heart Rate	Duration Intensity	Comments (e.g., rating of perceived exertion, pain, observations)
October 1	Walk/jog	60 to 70% of MHR	30 minutes	Great being outdoors

Date	Activity	Heart Rate	Duration Intensity	Comments (e.g., rating of perceived exertion, pain, observations)
October 1	Walk/jog	60 to 70% of MHR	30 minutes	Great being outdoors

Cardiorespiratory Endurance Training Log

Name: ——————————————————— Course Number: ———————————

Section: ——————————————— Date: ———————————————

Rockport Fitness Walking Test™

This activity assesses cardiorespiratory (aerobic) fitness. To perform the test, you need a watch with a second hand to record your time, and you need to wear good walking shoes and loose clothes. You should have answered NO to all the PAR-Q questions before taking this exercise test (see Activity 3.1).

Instructions

1. Find a measured track or measure 1 mile using your car's odometer on a level, uninterrupted road.

2. Warm up by walking slowly for 5 minutes.

3. Walk 1 mile as fast as you can, maintaining a steady pace. Note the time that you began walking.

4. When you complete the mile walk, record your time to the nearest second and keep walking at a slower pace. Count your pulse for 15 seconds and multiply by 4, and then record this number. This gives your heart rate per minute after your test walk.

Heart rate at the end of 1-mile walk: ———— beats per minute

Time to walk the mile: ———— minutes

5. Remember to stretch once you have cooled down.

6. To find your cardiorespiratory fitness level, refer to the appropriate Rockport Fitness Walking Test™ charts based on your age and sex. These show established fitness norms from the American Heart Association.

Using your fitness level chart, find your time in minutes and your heart rate per minute. Follow these lines until they meet, and mark this point on your chart. This tells you how fit you are compared to other individuals of your sex and age category.

These charts are based on weights of 170 lb for men and 125 lb for women. If you weigh substantially less, your cardiovascular fitness will be slightly underestimated. Conversely, if you weigh substantially more, your cardiovascular fitness will be slightly overestimated.

How fit you are compared to others of the same age and gender:

Level 5 = high
Level 4 = above average
Level 3 = average
Level 2 = below average
Level 1 = low

Find your fitness level using the Rockport Fitness Walking Test™.

MEN'S FITNESS LEVEL CHART

WOMEN'S FITNESS LEVEL CHART

AGE 20–29

AGE 30–39

AGE 40–49

AGE 50–59

AGE 60+

Source: The Rockport Company, LLC, © 1993. *The Rockport Company Walking Test.* The Rockport Company, LLC, Canton, MA. Reprinted with permission of The Rockport Company, LLC.

Results and Reflections

_____

_____

_____

_____

Chapter 4: Critical Thinking Questions

The Heart of Physical Fitness: Cardiorespiratory Endurance

1. In the vignette, Maria decided to use the heart rate reserve method to determine her aerobic exercise intensity. What other methods could she have utilized to determine her exercise intensity?

2. Identify four activities in which you are likely to participate that will enhance your cardiorespiratory endurance. Describe how you will incorporate each activity into your daily and weekly routine.

_____

_____

_____

_____

_____

_____

_____

_____

_____

_____

_____

_____

_____

_____

_____

_____

_____

Critical Thinking Questions

Name: _____ Course Number: _____

Section: _____ Date: _____

Resistance Exercise Readiness and Goal Setting

Directions: Indicate your stage of change in Step 1 and complete Steps 2, 3, 4, or 5, depending on which ones apply to your stage of change.

Step 1: Your Stage of Behavior Change

Please indicate which of the following statements best describes your readiness to follow the American College of Sports Medicine's recommendation for resistance exercise of performing "strength training or weight lifting exercises 2 to 3 days a week for each major muscle group."

_____ Description of the resistance exercise recommendation doesn't match my current behavior patterns, and I don't intend to change them to be like it in the next 6 months. (Precontemplation)

_____ Description of the resistance exercise recommendation doesn't match my current behavior patterns, but I do intend to change them to be like it in the next 6 months. (Contemplation)

_____ Description of the resistance exercise recommendation doesn't match my current behavior patterns, but I am motivated and confident that I can change them to be like it in the next month. (Preparation)

_____ Description of the resistance exercise recommendation is similar to my current behavior patterns, but I've been practicing this behavior for less than 6 months. (Action)

_____ Description of the resistance exercise recommendation is similar to my current behavior patterns, and I've been practicing this behavior for 6 months or longer. (Maintenance)

Step 2: Precontemplation or Contemplation

Your goal is to begin thinking about this exercise recommendation. You will consider the ways you could benefit from this behavior and think about how you could overcome any obstacles that are preventing you from practicing this behavior.

Imagine that a friend or family member was told by his or her health care provider to adopt this exercise recommendation. What advantages of this exercise recommendation would you highlight to motivate your friend or family member? (List at least three.)

_____

_____

What are some things that might get in the way of this person's efforts to implement this exercise recommendation? (List at least two.) What ideas do you have to help your friend or family member overcome these obstacles?

_____

_____

Now consider your own costs and benefits for adopting this exercise recommendation.

Reasons to Change	Reasons to Stay the Same
1. _____	1. _____
2. _____	2. _____
3. _____	3. _____
4. _____	4. _____
5. _____	5. _____

What one benefit of this exercise recommendation do you think will motivate you the most?

_____

_____

What one "cost" or barrier do you think will present the biggest obstacle for you?

_____

_____

Other people can help or hinder the behavior change process. Identify at least one person who can support your efforts, and list one or more things he or she can do to provide support.

_____

_____

Step 3: Preparation

Your goal is to commit to this exercise recommendation soon. You will do so by setting small, realistic goals and creating a plan to take action.

What changes will you need to make to achieve this exercise recommendation? In other words, what will you need to do differently to succeed?

_____

_____

Write one or two SMART goals that will help you achieve this exercise recommendation:

1. _____

2. _____

Commit to take action. Set a start date: _____

Tell someone what you plan to do. Being accountable to others motivates you and also offers you support and encouragement.

Who did you tell? _____

Signature: _____

Step 4: Action

Your goal is to firmly establish this behavior as a lifelong habit by anticipating problems and preparing to overcome failures, and by rewarding your success to stay committed.

Track your progress. For 7 days after your start date, keep track of the results of trying to meet your SMART goal(s) on the following chart:

SMART Goals	Dates	Results

Evaluate your progress and continue or modify your plan:

_____

_____

In what ways have you benefited from adopting this behavior?

_____

_____

What motivates you the most to continue practicing this behavior and why?

_____

_____

Reward your progress. Permanently changing lifestyle behaviors takes patience and consistent positive reinforcement. List several rewards you could give yourself for meeting your goals:

_____

_____

Select a reward for meeting your goal(s) for 7 days: _____

Select a reward for meeting your goal(s) for 1 month: _____

Step 5: Maintenance

Your goal is to stay focused and renew your commitment to this behavior. You will consider new ways to achieve your goals for long-term health and identify ways to prevent the inevitable slip-ups from becoming full-fledged backslides.

What benefits of practicing this exercise recommendation are most important to you, and why?

_____

_____

How easy is this exercise recommendation to maintain? Is it truly a habit or do you need to expend some effort to do it?

_____

_____

Sometimes you might get off track briefly (but hopefully not permanently) and need to recommit yourself to this exercise recommendation. How frequently do you not meet this exercise recommendation and why?

_____

_____

Name: _____ Course Number: _____

Section: _____ Date: _____

Experience Resistance Exercises

Directions: From the types of resistance exercises illustrated in Chapter 5 of *Physical Activity and Health, Fourth Edition*, select three exercises for each of the major muscle groups. You may list an exercise more than one time if it is a multi-joint exercise (works more than one muscle group). Next to each exercise you list, check whether or not you have actually performed the exercise in the last year.

Muscle Group	Exercises	Performed	
		Yes	No
Legs	1. 2. 3.		
Hips	1. 2. 3.		
Back	1. 2. 3.		
Chest	1. 2. 3.		
Abdomen	1. 2. 3.		
Shoulders	1. 2. 3.		
Arms	1. 2. 3.		

If you have not performed a resistance exercise you listed for a specific muscle group in the last year, are you willing to in the next 30 days? _____ Yes _____ No

Explain: _____

_____

If you performed resistance exercises on different muscle groups, what did you learn about your muscular strength and endurance levels in the different muscle groups?

_____

_____

If you performed multiple resistance exercises for the same muscle group, which exercise did you prefer and why?

_____

_____

Name: _____   Course Number: _____

Section: _____   Date: _____

Resistance Training Log

Directions: Track and record your resistance exercise progress by date, sets, reps, and weight.

Sample of Resistance Exercises

Muscle Group	Training with Weights (free weights or resistance machines)	Without Weights
Chest	Bench press	Push-ups; modified push-ups
Shoulder	Shoulder press	Pull-ups, chin-ups, modified dips
Arm (bicep)	Bicep curl	Arm curl, chin-ups
Arm (tricep)	Tricep curl	Pull-ups, modified dips
Hip/leg	Lunges	Lunges
Leg (thigh)	Half squat	
Leg (calf)	Heel raise	Heel raise

Monitor your workouts by recording the number of sets, repetitions, and the amount of weight.

Muscle group exercises	Date: set × rep / wt	Date: set × rep / wt	Date: set × rep / wt	Date: set × rep / wt	Date: set × rep / wt
	× /	× /	× /	× /	× /
	× /	× /	× /	× /	× /
	× /	× /	× /	× /	× /
	× /	× /	× /	× /	× /
	× /	× /	× /	× /	× /
	× /	× /	× /	× /	× /
	× /	× /	× /	× /	× /
	× /	× /	× /	× /	× /
	× /	× /	× /	× /	× /
	× /	× /	× /	× /	× /

Muscle group exercises	Date: set × rep / wt	Date: set × rep / wt	Date: set × rep / wt	Date: set × rep / wt	Date: set × rep / wt
	× /	× /	× /	× /	× /
	× /	× /	× /	× /	× /
	× /	× /	× /	× /	× /
	× /	× /	× /	× /	× /
	× /	× /	× /	× /	× /
	× /	× /	× /	× /	× /
	× /	× /	× /	× /	× /
	× /	× /	× /	× /	× /
	× /	× /	× /	× /	× /
	× /	× /	× /	× /	× /

Muscle group exercises	Date: set × rep / wt	Date: set × rep / wt	Date: set × rep / wt	Date: set × rep / wt	Date: set × rep / wt
	× /	× /	× /	× /	× /
	× /	× /	× /	× /	× /
	× /	× /	× /	× /	× /
	× /	× /	× /	× /	× /
	× /	× /	× /	× /	× /
	× /	× /	× /	× /	× /
	× /	× /	× /	× /	× /
	× /	× /	× /	× /	× /
	× /	× /	× /	× /	× /
	× /	× /	× /	× /	× /

Name: _____   Course Number: _____

Section: _____   Date: _____

Measuring Muscular Endurance

Many muscular endurance fitness tests require special equipment or a professionally trained exercise specialist to administer the test—however not all do. The following three tests are designed to quickly gauge a person's general muscular endurance level with minimal equipment. Each is safe to perform providing you do not have injuries or pain that could be worsened by a specific movement (e.g., doing pushups with shoulder or elbow pain) and you answered NO to all the PAR-Q questions (Activity 3.1).

Directions: Simple descriptions of each muscular endurance test are provided. Wear loose comfortable clothes and athletic shoes. Do each test with plenty of rest between so that you are fully recovered. Do a warm-up first. A general warm-up procedure for your testing is to walk briskly for 5 to 10 minutes. The tests are listed in recommended order.

1. **Push-up Test: Assesses endurance of the chest, shoulder, and triceps muscles.** Assume the standard position for a push-up, with the body rigid and straight, toes tucked under, and hands about shoulderwidth apart and directly under the shoulders. Lower the body until the elbows reach 90 degrees. Return to the starting position with arms fully extended. Do not hold your breath during the exertion phase. Females can modify the standard position by having their knees touch the floor. Complete as many push-ups as you can in 1 minute, or until failure without any break in proper form.

   Record your number of push-ups _____.

2. **Crunches or Half Sit-Up Test: Assesses endurance of the abdominal and hip flexor muscles.** Lie on a carpeted floor or an exercise mat. Assume the starting position for a crunch with bent knees at approximately 90-degree angles, feet flat on the floor, and hands resting on your thighs. Slide your hands along your thighs until your fingers touch the top of your knees while keeping your lower back on the floor. Do not hold your breath during the exertion phase. Return to the starting position. Do not pull with your neck or head. Complete as many crunches as you can in 1 minute, or until failure without any break in proper form.

   Record your number of half sit-ups _____.

3. **Chair Stand Test: Assesses endurance of the quadriceps muscle.** Stand in front of a chair with your feet shoulderwidth apart, facing away from it. Place your hands on your hips. Squat down as if you are going to take a seat in the chair. Lightly touch the chair with your butt before standing back up. Keep your weight on your heels

and do not let your knees shoot past your toes. Select a chair size that allows your knees to bend at 90-degree angles when you are sitting. Do not hold your breath during the exertion phase. Complete as many squats as you can in 1 minute, or until failure without any break in proper form.

Record your number of chair stands ——————.

How to Use Your Test Results

Use the results as a benchmark for future testing. Set fitness goals based on what you've learned. For example, you may want to set a goal of being able to perform 5 more push-ups the next time you complete the test. Give yourself 4 to 6 weeks of regular resistance training to allow for improvements before taking a test again. You should see some progress in your muscular endurance scores.

Chapter 5: Critical Thinking Questions

The Power of Resistance Training: Strengthening Your Health

1. List five ways resistance training improves your health.

2. Explain the sliding filament theory of muscle contraction.

3. Explain two differences between slow-twitch and fast-twitch muscle fibers.

4. Explain the differences between static and dynamic resistance-type exercises.

5. Explain the FITT principle as it applies to a resistance training program.

———

———

———

———

———

———

———

———

———

———

———

———

———

———

———

———

———

———

———

———

———

Critical Thinking Questions

Name: _____ Course Number: _____

Section: _____ Date: _____

Flexibility Exercise Readiness and Goal Setting

Directions: Indicate your stage of change in Step 1 and complete Steps 2, 3, 4, or 5, depending on which ones apply to your stage of change.

Step 1: Your Stage of Behavior Change

Please indicate which of the following statements best describes your readiness to follow the American College of Sports Medicine's recommendation for flexibility exercise of performing "a series of stretching exercises for each major muscle-tendon group (a total of 60 seconds per exercise) on 2 or more days a week."

_____ Description of the flexibility exercise recommendation doesn't match my current behavior patterns, and I don't intend to change them to be like it in the next 6 months. (Precontemplation)

_____ Description of the flexibility exercise recommendation doesn't match my current behavior patterns, but I do intend to change them to be like it in the next 6 months. (Contemplation)

_____ Description of the flexibility exercise recommendation doesn't match my current behavior patterns, but I am motivated and confident that I can change them to be like it in the next month. (Preparation)

_____ Description of the flexibility exercise recommendation is similar to my current behavior patterns, but I've been practicing this behavior for less than 6 months. (Action)

_____ Description of the flexibility exercise recommendation is similar to my current behavior patterns, and I've been practicing this behavior for 6 months or longer. (Maintenance)

Step 2: Precontemplation or Contemplation

Your goal is to begin thinking about this exercise recommendation. You will consider the ways you could benefit from this behavior and think about how you could overcome any obstacles that are preventing you from practicing this behavior.

Imagine that a friend or family member was told by his or her health care provider to adopt this exercise recommendation. What advantages of this exercise recommendation would you highlight to motivate your friend or family member? (List at least three.)

_____

_____

What are some things that might get in the way of this person's efforts to implement this exercise recommendation? (List at least two.) What ideas do you have to help your friend or family member overcome these obstacles?

_____

_____

Now consider your own costs and benefits for adopting this exercise recommendation.

Reasons to Change	Reasons to Stay the Same
1. _____	1. _____
2. _____	2. _____
3. _____	3. _____
4. _____	4. _____
5. _____	5. _____

What one benefit of this exercise recommendation do you think will motivate you the most?

_____

_____

What one "cost" or barrier do you think will present the biggest obstacle for you?

_____

_____

Other people can help or hinder the behavior change process. Identify at least one person who can support your efforts, and list one or more things he or she can do to provide support.

_____

_____

Step 3: Preparation

Your goal is to commit to this exercise recommendation soon. You will do so by setting small, realistic goals and creating a plan to take action.

What changes will you need to make to achieve this exercise recommendation? In other words, what will you need to do differently to succeed?

_____

_____

Write one or two SMART goals that will help you achieve this exercise recommendation:

1. _____

2. _____

Commit to take action. Set a start date: _____

Tell someone what you plan to do. Being accountable to others motivates you and also offers you support and encouragement.

Who did you tell? _____

Signature: _____

Step 4: Action

Your goal is to firmly establish this behavior as a lifelong habit by anticipating problems and preparing to overcome failures, and by rewarding your success to stay committed.

Track your progress. For 7 days after your start date, keep track of the results of trying to meet your SMART goal(s) on the following chart:

SMART Goals	Dates	Results

Evaluate your progress and continue or modify your plan:

_____

_____

In what ways have you benefited from adopting this behavior?

_____

_____

What motivates you the most to continue practicing this behavior, and why?

_____

_____

Reward your progress. Permanently changing lifestyle behaviors takes patience and consistent positive reinforcement. List several rewards you could give yourself for meeting your goals:

_____

_____

Select a reward for meeting your goal(s) for 7 days: _____

Select a reward for meeting your goal(s) for 1 month: _____

Step 5: Maintenance

Your goal is to stay focused and renew your commitment to this behavior. You will consider new ways to achieve your goals for long-term health and identify ways to prevent the inevitable slip-ups from becoming full-fledged backslides.

What benefits of practicing this exercise recommendation are most important to you, and why?

_____

_____

How easy is this exercise recommendation to maintain? Is it truly a habit or do you need to expend some effort to do it?

_____

_____

Sometimes you might get off track briefly (but hopefully not permanently) and need to recommit yourself to this exercise recommendation. How frequently do you not meet this exercise recommendation and why?

_____

_____

Name: _____ Course Number: _____

Section: _____ Date: _____

Experience Flexibility Exercises

Sample Stretching Program

Upper Body/Torso Stretching

Stretch	Figure	Area of Proposed Stretch	Secondary Stretch Location
1 Ear to shoulder left and right	6.6	Neck lateral flexion	
2 Chin to chest and chin raised	6.7	Neck flexion and extension	
3 Look right and left	6.8	Neck stretch	

Note: Perform the above neck-stretching exercises in circuit format. Neck rotations are not advised.

Stretch	Figure	Area of Proposed Stretch	Secondary Stretch Location
4 Arm across chest	6.9	Rear shoulder and arm	
5 Shoulder girdle stretch	6.10	Front shoulder and chest	
6 Handcuff stretch	6.11	Shoulders, chest, and upper back	
7 Overhead triceps	6.12	Upper arms and shoulders	
8 Seated side reach	6.13	Back and shoulders	
9 Bent over lat stretch	6.14	Back and shoulders	
10 Prone torso extension	6.15	Lower back and shoulders	

Lower Body/Torso Stretching

Stretch	Figure	Area of Proposed Stretch	Secondary Stretch Location
1 Elbow to knee	6.16	Gluteal and lower trunk	
2 Modified hurdler	6.17	Hamstring, lower back, and groin	
3 Lying iliotibial stretch	6.18	Quadricep and hip	
4 Side-lying infraspinatus stretch	6.19	Quadricep and hip	
5 Kneeling stretch	6.20	Lower back and hip flexor	
6 Standing heel to buttocks	6.21	Quadricep	
7 Lunging hip flexor stretch	6.22	Quadricep and hip flexor	
8 Prone glute stretch	6.23	Glute and lower back	
9 Hip abductors stretch	6.24	Hip abductors	
10 Wall lean	6.25	Calf	
11 Seated shin stretch	6.26	Shin	

All stretching activities should be preceded by a 5–10 minute warm-up period consisting of large muscle group activity. It is recommended that all static stretches be held for 15 to 60 seconds. Do not hold your breath at any time during a stretch. Exercises that stretch the major muscle groups should be performed a minimum of 2 to 3 days a week.

Note: It is suitable to stretch the upper body one day and the lower body the next.

Note: It is advisable to take note of where the stretching exercise is felt. Even though the primary function of the muscle stretch may be felt, pay close attention to secondary stretch locations in other areas. Chart these areas because this is a sign of tightness in other areas, which should be addressed for balance.

Directions: Select three upper body and three lower body stretches to perform. Each of the stretches are illustrated in Chapter 6. Hold each stretch for 10 to 30 seconds and repeat twice. Do not hold your breath. Wear loose, comfortable clothes. Do a warm-up first. A general warm-up procedure before you begin stretching is to walk briskly for 5 to 10 minutes.

What are two things you learned from completing these stretching exercises?

_____

_____

What did you learn about your upper body and lower body flexibility?

_____

_____

If you performed multiple stretching exercises for the same muscle group, which exercise did you prefer and why?

_____

_____

Name: _____ Course Number: _____

Section: _____ Date: _____

Stretching Log

Step 1: Select stretching exercises and write them in the left column.

Step 2: Circle the days of each week you stretched.

Exercise	Week of	Week of	Week of
	S M T W Th F Sa	S M T W Th F Sa	S M T W Th F Sa
	S M T W Th F Sa	S M T W Th F Sa	S M T W Th F Sa
	S M T W Th F Sa	S M T W Th F Sa	S M T W Th F Sa
	S M T W Th F Sa	S M T W Th F Sa	S M T W Th F Sa
	S M T W Th F Sa	S M T W Th F Sa	S M T W Th F Sa
	S M T W Th F Sa	S M T W Th F Sa	S M T W Th F Sa
	S M T W Th F Sa	S M T W Th F Sa	S M T W Th F Sa
	S M T W Th F Sa	S M T W Th F Sa	S M T W Th F Sa
	S M T W Th F Sa	S M T W Th F Sa	S M T W Th F Sa
	S M T W Th F Sa	S M T W Th F Sa	S M T W Th F Sa
	S M T W Th F Sa	S M T W Th F Sa	S M T W Th F Sa
	S M T W Th F Sa	S M T W Th F Sa	S M T W Th F Sa

Exercise	Week of	Week of	Week of
	S M T W Th F Sa	S M T W Th F Sa	S M T W Th F Sa
	S M T W Th F Sa	S M T W Th F Sa	S M T W Th F Sa
	S M T W Th F Sa	S M T W Th F Sa	S M T W Th F Sa
	S M T W Th F Sa	S M T W Th F Sa	S M T W Th F Sa
	S M T W Th F Sa	S M T W Th F Sa	S M T W Th F Sa
	S M T W Th F Sa	S M T W Th F Sa	S M T W Th F Sa
	S M T W Th F Sa	S M T W Th F Sa	S M T W Th F Sa
	S M T W Th F Sa	S M T W Th F Sa	S M T W Th F Sa
	S M T W Th F Sa	S M T W Th F Sa	S M T W Th F Sa
	S M T W Th F Sa	S M T W Th F Sa	S M T W Th F Sa
	S M T W Th F Sa	S M T W Th F Sa	S M T W Th F Sa
	S M T W Th F Sa	S M T W Th F Sa	S M T W Th F Sa

Exercise	Week of	Week of	Week of
	S M T W Th F Sa	S M T W Th F Sa	S M T W Th F Sa
	S M T W Th F Sa	S M T W Th F Sa	S M T W Th F Sa
	S M T W Th F Sa	S M T W Th F Sa	S M T W Th F Sa
	S M T W Th F Sa	S M T W Th F Sa	S M T W Th F Sa
	S M T W Th F Sa	S M T W Th F Sa	S M T W Th F Sa
	S M T W Th F Sa	S M T W Th F Sa	S M T W Th F Sa
	S M T W Th F Sa	S M T W Th F Sa	S M T W Th F Sa
	S M T W Th F Sa	S M T W Th F Sa	S M T W Th F Sa
	S M T W Th F Sa	S M T W Th F Sa	S M T W Th F Sa
	S M T W Th F Sa	S M T W Th F Sa	S M T W Th F Sa
	S M T W Th F Sa	S M T W Th F Sa	S M T W Th F Sa
	S M T W Th F Sa	S M T W Th F Sa	S M T W Th F Sa

Exercise	Week of	Week of	Week of
	S M T W Th F Sa	S M T W Th F Sa	S M T W Th F Sa
	S M T W Th F Sa	S M T W Th F Sa	S M T W Th F Sa
	S M T W Th F Sa	S M T W Th F Sa	S M T W Th F Sa
	S M T W Th F Sa	S M T W Th F Sa	S M T W Th F Sa
	S M T W Th F Sa	S M T W Th F Sa	S M T W Th F Sa
	S M T W Th F Sa	S M T W Th F Sa	S M T W Th F Sa
	S M T W Th F Sa	S M T W Th F Sa	S M T W Th F Sa
	S M T W Th F Sa	S M T W Th F Sa	S M T W Th F Sa
	S M T W Th F Sa	S M T W Th F Sa	S M T W Th F Sa
	S M T W Th F Sa	S M T W Th F Sa	S M T W Th F Sa
	S M T W Th F Sa	S M T W Th F Sa	S M T W Th F Sa
	S M T W Th F Sa	S M T W Th F Sa	S M T W Th F Sa

Exercise	Week of	Week of	Week of
	S M T W Th F Sa	S M T W Th F Sa	S M T W Th F Sa
	S M T W Th F Sa	S M T W Th F Sa	S M T W Th F Sa
	S M T W Th F Sa	S M T W Th F Sa	S M T W Th F Sa
	S M T W Th F Sa	S M T W Th F Sa	S M T W Th F Sa
	S M T W Th F Sa	S M T W Th F Sa	S M T W Th F Sa
	S M T W Th F Sa	S M T W Th F Sa	S M T W Th F Sa
	S M T W Th F Sa	S M T W Th F Sa	S M T W Th F Sa
	S M T W Th F Sa	S M T W Th F Sa	S M T W Th F Sa
	S M T W Th F Sa	S M T W Th F Sa	S M T W Th F Sa
	S M T W Th F Sa	S M T W Th F Sa	S M T W Th F Sa
	S M T W Th F Sa	S M T W Th F Sa	S M T W Th F Sa
	S M T W Th F Sa	S M T W Th F Sa	S M T W Th F Sa

Name: _____ Course Number: _____

Section: _____ Date: _____

Sit-and-Reach Test

Precautions

1. Warm up.

2. Stop the test if pain occurs.

3. Do not be competitive. Do not perform fast, jerky movements.

4. If any of the following apply, seek medical advice before performing tests:

   a. You are presently suffering from acute back pain.

   b. You are currently receiving treatment for back pain.

   c. You have ever had a surgical operation on your back.

   d. A health care professional told you to never exercise your back.

Procedure

Step 1

Sit on the floor with your legs straight, knees together, and toes pointing upward toward the ceiling.

Step 2

Place one hand over the other. The tips of your two middle fingers should be on top of each other. Slowly stretch forward without bouncing or jerking. Stop when tightness or discomfort occurs in the back or legs.

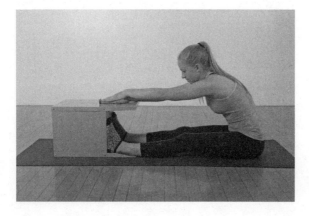

Step 3

Repeat this test two more times and record scores.

First attempt   —————— points

Second attempt   —————— points

Third attempt   —————— points

How to score (average of 3 attempts):

Reached well past toes	1 point; excellent
Reached just to toes	2 points; good
Up to 4 inches from toes	3 points; fair
More than 4 inches from toes	4 points; poor

Source: Reproduced from David Imrie. (1988). *Back Power.* Toronto, Canada: Stoddart, 83. Courtesy of David Imrie.

Total points = —————— divided by 3 = —————— points, which is rated as ——————.

Chapter 6: Critical Thinking Questions

Focus on Flexibility: Stretching for Better Health

1. The health benefits of being flexible—the ability to move a joint through its complete range of motion—are many. List three health benefits and how each could enhance your quality of life.

2. Based on your current flexibility program and time commitments, identify three different types of stretching exercises and briefly explain which type you would prefer and why.

3. Many factors influence the amount of flexibility you have at a joint. List two factors over which you have control and whether or not you have taken action on these factors.

_____

_____

_____

_____

_____

_____

_____

_____

_____

_____

_____

_____

_____

_____

Critical Thinking Questions

Name: _____ Course Number: _____

Section: _____ Date: _____

Diet and Activity Records

Worksheets are provided in Appendix A of this manual to record your dietary intake and your activities. Select a combination of weekdays and weekend days according to your instructor's directions. Use a new record for each day. The worksheets have been labeled accordingly. Be sure to fill in your name and the date and indicate whether it was a weekday or weekend day at the top of each record. The idea is to get a representative record of intake and expenditure on both typical "workdays" and typical "leisure days." Each day, fill in *both* a diet record and an activity record. This step is important for comparing energy intake and expenditure.

It is essential for you to be complete, accurate, and honest in your record keeping. If the information you record is fictional or inaccurate, you will not learn anything personally valuable from your analysis, and the hours you spend on this effort will be a waste of time. You do not get a better grade for "healthier" habits, so don't fake the information to "look better." Take the records with you and log information continuously throughout the day rather than waiting until the end of the day and relying on your memory. Keep track of *everything* you consume and *everything* you do, accurately listing the amounts and times. Using a pencil will allow you to correct mistakes, but be sure it writes dark enough to be readable and photocopy well.

Directions for Completing the Diet Records

The diet record is quite detailed, but the information will prove very useful when you analyze your eating behaviors, and much of the information is recorded only once for each eating event. Each time an eating event occurs, whether it is a meal, a snack, or the consumption of a beverage, record the following information as indicated on the sample diet record:

- What time of day it was, including whether it was a.m. or p.m.

- Whether the event was a meal (M), a snack (S), or a beverage (B).

- How hungry or thirsty you were (record in the column labeled "H"); see the rating scale at the bottom of the worksheet.

- Where you were, such as a cafeteria, restaurant, kitchen table, bedroom, or car (record in the column labeled "Location," and be as specific as you can).

- Whether you were doing any activity while eating (such as driving, watching TV, studying, or talking on the phone).

- If others were present, who (roommates, spouse, friends, and so on), or else write "alone."

- How much time was spent eating/drinking (record in minutes)?

All of this information should be recorded only once for each eating event.

Recording Your Food and Beverage Intake

- In the column labeled "Food Eaten and Quantity," record each food and beverage you consumed on a separate line.

- Measure and record the amounts *eaten* using standard units of measurement (e.g., cups, teaspoons, tablespoons, ounces, size of food). The amount you record is the amount you *ate*, not necessarily the amount you were served. *Accurate measurement is critical for your assessment to be valid.*

- Be specific about brand names, types or varieties of food, and preparation (e.g., *Pepperidge Farm whole wheat* bread, *cheddar* cheese, *1%* milk, *Del Monte canned* pineapple *in heavy syrup*).

- Don't forget to list extras such as condiments, dressings, gravies, and sauces.

- Record all beverages consumed, including water.

- Record any dietary supplements taken. (You will *not* enter this information into your computer analysis, but will analyze it separately.)

For combination foods, list the components on separate lines.

For example, instead of "1 turkey sub," write 12-inch wheat sub bun, 6 1-ounce slices turkey, 3 leaves lettuce, 3 slices tomato, 2 tablespoons mayonnaise.

Picturing Portions

A *portion* is the amount of food you actually eat. It may be more or less than the standard *serving*, which is the amount listed on food labels and the reference amount listed in food composition tables. As much as possible, measure your food when you keep your diet records. When that is not possible, you can compare the size or amount to common objects:

A *medium* potato is the size of a computer mouse.

A *medium-size* fruit or vegetable is the size of your clenched fist or a tennis ball.

One-half cup of rice, pasta, cereal, or chopped vegetables or fruit is a rounded handful.

One-fourth cup of dried fruit or raisins is the size of a golf ball.

An *average* bagel is the size of a hockey puck.

A pancake or a slice of bread is the size of a CD.

A *cup* of fruit is the size of a baseball.

A *cup* of lettuce is four leaves.

Three ounces of cooked meat or poultry is the size of a deck of cards.

Three ounces of grilled fish is the size of your palm.

One ounce of cheese is the size of four dice or two dominoes.

One teaspoon of butter or margarine is the size of a postage stamp.

One tablespoon of salad dressing is the size of a thumb tip.

Two tablespoons of peanut butter is the size of a Ping-Pong ball.

One cup of cooked dry beans is the size of a tennis ball.

One ounce of nuts or small candies is one small handful.

One ounce of chips or pretzels is a large handful.

Recording Measures of Motivators to Eat, Eating More/Less Than Served, and Termination of Eating

- In the column labeled "Reason for Choice," describe *why* you chose each food. Some possible reasons are listed at the bottom of the worksheet, but many others exist.

- Indicate in the column labeled "Helpings" whether you ate less than (−), equal to (0), or more than (+) your *original* helping of that food/beverage.

> *The amount of food recorded in the "Food Eaten and Quantity" column should be the amount eaten, not the amount served. For example, if you measured out one cup, but ate only three-fourths of a cup, list 3/4 cup in the "Food Eaten" column and designate that less was eaten than was served by putting a minus sign (−) in the "Helpings" column.*

- The final column, labeled "S," should be filled in only once at the end of each eating event. Indicate your degree of satiation (fullness) using the rating scale provided at the bottom of the worksheet.

Directions for Completing the Activity Records

Record your activities on the same days you keep your diet records. Worksheets are labeled day 1, day 2, day 3, and so on, for this purpose. Be sure to record your name and the date, and indicate whether it was a weekday or weekend day at the top of each worksheet.

- Begin each day with 12 a.m. (midnight) and end with the following midnight.

- Every time you change from one activity to another, record the time you ended the previous activity and started the new one, and describe the type of activity.

- Break down your activity record so that each line is consecutive to cover the 1440 minutes in 24 hours.

- Each time your activity changes, make a new entry.

- Periodically throughout the day, or at the end of the day, fill in the duration and the level of activity columns.

- Record duration in minutes. For example, if you slept from midnight to 7:15 a.m., record 435 minutes.

- At the end of 24 hours, the total time you have recorded must equal 1440 minutes.

You can use the following table to determine your "level of activity." Similar activities have very similar energy expenditures, so they can be grouped together on your activity record if they occurred in the same time period (e.g., reading and typing as part of "studying").

Although activities such as playing computer games or watching television use the same amount of energy as studying, list these activities separately on your activity record so that you have an accurate reflection of how you spend your time. In other words, if you are watching TV and studying at the same time, determine how much time you are doing each activity and record them accordingly. If in your assessment you determine that you are more sedentary than your energy intake allows for, it would be better to cut back on time spent watching TV or playing computer games than on time spent studying.

Basal Metabolism The energy cost of staying alive (e.g., sleeping, lying motionless).

Sedentary (0.01 kcal/min/kg) Sitting with little or no body movements (e.g., reading, writing, eating, watching television, driving, sewing).

Light (0.02 kcal/min/kg) Sitting or standing with some movement of arms and other parts of the body (e.g., preparing food, dish-washing, walking at 2 mi/h, bathing).

Moderate (0.03 kcal/min/kg) Sitting with vigorous arm movements, or standing with considerable movement (e.g., making beds, mopping, walking at 4 mi/h, warm-up and cooldown exercises, bowling, golfing).

Vigorous (0.06 kcal/min/kg) Moving body rapidly (e.g., tennis, jogging, weight-lifting, team sports—basketball, baseball, football—but only while playing).

Strenuous (0.10 kcal/min/kg) Moving body at maximum or near maximum capacity (e.g., swimming laps, running, rope jumping). This level is aerobic activity. Do not include warm-up and cooldown periods.

Examples of diet and activity records are provided on the following pages.

Diet Record Day 1

Name: _____ Date: _____

☐ Weekday
☐ Weekend Day

Sample

Eating Behavior Diary

Time of Day	M, S, or B[1]	H[2] (0–3)	Location	Activity While Eating	Others Present	Time Spent Eating	Food Eaten and Quantity (describe preparation, variety, etc., as needed)	Reason for Choice[3]	Helpings (0,–,+)[4]	S[5] (0–3)
7:45 a.m.	M	2	Dining hall	Visiting	Friends	15 min	6 ounces orange juice	Health	0	2
							1 cup Cheerios	Health, habit	–	
							3/4 cup 2% milk	Health, habit	–	
							1/2 toasted bagel	Taste	0	
							1 Tbsp cream cheese	Taste	0	
9:30 a.m.	B	1	Union	Studying	Alone	30	16-ounce Coke	Caffeine	0	2
11:35 a.m.	M	2	McDonald's	Reading paper	Alone	20	Quarter Pounder with cheese	Taste	–	3
							Large French fry	Comfort	0	
							Large Coke	Caffeine	–	
4:15 p.m.	B	2	Swimming pool	Changing clothes	Alone	10	1/2 of 16-ounce water bottle	Thirsty	0	1
5:00 p.m.	B	2	Swimming pool	Changing clothes	Alone	10	1/2 of 16-ounce water bottle	Thirsty	0	1
5:50 p.m.	M	2	Dining hall	Visiting	Friends	30	12 ounces 2% milk	Health, habit	0	2
							12 ounces water	Health	0	
							1 cup tossed salad	Health	0	
							1 ounce grated cheese	Taste, health	0	
							2 Tbsp ranch dressing	Taste	0	

[1] Indicate whether the eating/drinking event was a meal, a snack, or a beverage.

[2] Degree of hunger: 0 = not at all hungry; 1 = slightly hungry; 2 = moderately hungry; 3 = very hungry. If only a beverage was consumed, apply the scale to the degree of thirst.

[3] Reason for food choice: Examples include taste, habit, convenience, health, weight control, hunger, thirst, stress, comfort, offered to me, and so on.

[4] Helpings: 0 = ate all that you were first served but not more; – = ate less than what you were served; + = ate more than you were originally served.

[5] Degree of satiation: 0 = not at all satisfied; 1 = still a little hungry; 2 = satisfied and comfortable; 3 = very full.

(continues)

Eating Behavior Diary

Time of Day	M, S, or B[1]	H[2] (0–3)	Location	Activity While Eating	Others Present	Time Spent Eating	Food Eaten and Quantity (describe preparation, variety, etc., as needed)	Reason for Choice[3]	Helpings (0,–,+)[4]	S[5] (0–3)
							3" × 3" square of lasagna:	Taste, health	0	
							1.5 ounces lasagna noodles, cooked			
							1 ounce cooked ground beef			
							1.5 ounces cottage cheese			
							4 ounces pasta sauce			
							1 ounce grated mozzarella cheese			
							2 slices garlic bread	Taste, habit	+	
							1 cup soft-serve ice cream	Taste	+	
10 p.m.	S	1	Dorm room	Studying	Alone	5 min	Snickers bar	Taste, habit	0	2
							16-ounce bottle fruit punch	Taste	0	

[1] Indicate whether the eating/drinking event was a meal, a snack, or a beverage.

[2] Degree of hunger: 0 = not at all hungry; 1 = slightly hungry; 2 = moderately hungry; 3 = very hungry. If only a beverage was consumed, apply the scale to the degree of thirst.

[3] Reason for food choice: Examples include taste, habit, convenience, health, weight control, hunger, thirst, stress, comfort, offered to me, and so on.

[4] Helpings: 0 = ate all that you were first served but not more; – = ate less than what you were served; + = ate more than you were originally served.

[5] Degree of satiation: 0 = not at all satisfied; 1 = still a little hungry; 2 = satisfied and comfortable; 3 = very full.

Activity Record Day 1

Name: _____*Sample*_____   Date: _____

☐ Weekday
☐ Weekend Day

Activity Record

Time of Day	Duration (Minutes)	Description of Activity	Level of Activity
12 – 7:15 a.m.	435	sleeping	basal
7:15 – 7:30	15	showering	light
7:30 – 7:40	10	dressing	light
7:40 – 7:45	5	walking	light
7:45 – 8:00	15	eating breakfast	sedentary
8:00 – 8:15	15	getting ready for class	light
8:15 – 8:30	15	walking to class	moderate
8:30 – 9:20	50	sitting in class	sedentary
9:20 – 9:30	10	walking to Union	moderate
9:30 – 10:20	50	sitting, reading	sedentary
10:20 – 10:30	10	walking to class	moderate
10:30 – 11:20	50	sitting in class	sedentary
11:20 – 11:35	15	walking to McDonald's	moderate
11:35 – 11:55	20	eating lunch	sedentary
11:55 – 12:00	5	walking to store	moderate
12:00 – 12:20	20	shopping for supplies	light
12:20 – 12:30	10	walking to library	moderate
12:30 – 2:20	110	studying	sedentary
2:20 – 2:30	10	walking to class	moderate
2:30 – 3:20	50	sitting in class	sedentary
3:20 – 3:35	15	walking to dorm	moderate
3:35 – 4:00	25	reading mail	sedentary
4:00 – 4:05	5	getting ready to swim	light
4:05 – 4:15	10	walking to swimming pool	moderate
4:15 – 4:25	10	change clothes, shower	light
4:25 – 4:30	5	warm-up swim	moderate
4:30 – 4:50	20	swim laps	strenuous
4:50 – 4:55	5	cooldown swim	moderate

Activity Record

Time of Day	Duration (Minutes)	Description of Activity	Level of Activity
4:55 – 5:15	20	shower and dress	light
5:15 – 5:25	10	walking to dorm	moderate
5:25 – 5:45	20	stand and talk to friends	light
5:45 – 5:50	5	walk to cafeteria	moderate
5:50 – 6:20	30	eat supper	sedentary
6:20 – 7:00	40	read e-mail, surf Internet	sedentary
7:00 – 7:45	45	watch television	sedentary
7:45 – 8:00	15	walk to study session	moderate
8:00 – 9:00	60	attend study session	sedentary
9:00 – 9:15	15	walk to dorm	moderate
9:15 – 11:00	105	studying	sedentary
11:00 – 11:15	15	getting ready for bed	light
11:15 – 12:00	45	sleeping	basal

Total Duration: 1440   (must equal 1440 minutes for the entire 24-hour period)

Name: ——————————————————————— Course Number: ———————————

Section: ——————————————————————— Date: ———————————————

SuperTracker Diet and Activity Analysis

The USDA's Center for Nutrition Policy and Promotion offers SuperTracker, a free online interactive tool for personalized diet and physical activity planning, assessment, and analysis. SuperTracker also provides personalized functions such as goal setting, virtual coaching, weight tracking and journaling, and individual customization for specific audiences and social networking integration. You can access SuperTracker by going to the website: https//www.supertracker.usda.gov. The SuperTracker Home page is shown here.

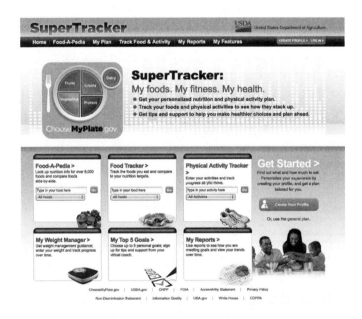

Source: Reproduced from The Center for Nutrition Policy and Promotion. U.S. Department of Agriculture. Online: https://www.supertracker.usda.gov.

Self-Assessment Activities:

1. **Create a Profile.** To get a diet and activity plan tailored for you, you need to create a profile by entering information about yourself. Click on "Create Profile." You will be asked to enter your name, age, gender, physical activity level, height, and weight. Register to save your information so that you can access it at any time.

2. **Get Your Plan.** View **My Plan** to see your daily food group targets. Your targets, based on your profile information, indicate what and how much you can eat within your calorie allowance. Save or print a copy for your reference.

3. **Track Your Foods.** To compare your daily food intake with your recommended intake in each food group from My Plan, click on "Food Tracker." Follow the online directions to assess your food intake. Enter your food intake for each 24-hour period you recorded using your completed diet record(s) from Activity 7.1. When you have entered all of your foods, you can analyze your food intake for each day by clicking "My Reports" and then "Nutrients Reports." Export the "Nutrients Reports" as a PDF. You will use the "Nutrients Reports" to answer the self-analysis questions as well as to compare your intake to your recommended nutrient intakes, the 2010 *Dietary Guidelines*, MyPlate recommendations, and your healthy eating history.

4. **Food Groups and Calories.** To obtain your average intake of calories and food groups for any period of time click on "My Reports" and then click "Food Groups & Calories." Export the "Food Groups & Calories Report" as a PDF file. You can compare your intake with the MyPlate recommendations.

5. **Track Your Activities.** To compare your daily physical activity with your recommended physical activity requirements, click on the "Physical Activity Tracker." Follow the online directions to assess your physical activity. Enter your activities for each 24-hour period you recorded on your activity record(s) from Activity 7.1. When you have entered all of your activities, you can analyze physical activity for each week by clicking on "Physical Activity Report." Export the report as a PDF. You can then view your weekly physical activities and compare them to the physical activity guidelines.

Self-Analysis:

1. Using your Nutrients Reports, what was your total caloric intake? _____ . Was the average number of calories you ate daily in the acceptable range? _____

   Explain: _____

2. Using your Nutrients Reports, what percent of your calories came from protein? _____ carbohydrates? _____ total fat? _____

3. Using your Nutrients Reports, how many of the nutrients were in the acceptable range? _____

   List them: _____

4. How many of the nutrients were not in the acceptable range? _____

   List them: _____

5. Was this day's food intake typical of other days? Yes ____ No ____

   Explain: _____

6. From the Food Groups & Calories Report complete this table:

Food Groups	Target	Average Eaten	Status
Grains			
Whole grains			
Refined grains			
Vegetables			
Dark green			
Red and orange			
Beans and peas			
Starchy			
Other			
Fruits			
Fruit juice			
Whole fruit			
Dairy			
Milk and yogurt			
Cheese			
Protein Foods			
Seafood			
Meat, poultry, and eggs			
Nuts, seeds, and soy			
Oils			
Limits	**Allowance**	**Average Eaten**	**Status**
Total calories			
Empty calories			
Solid fats			
Added sugars			

7. How many Food Groups were in the acceptable range? _____

   List them: _____

8. How many Food Groups were not in the acceptable range? _____

   List them: _____

9. Identify one action you can take to improve your food choices.

   Describe: _____

10. Using your Physical Activity Report, did you meet the *Physical Activity Guidelines for Americans* recommendations?

    Describe: _____

Name: _____ Course Number: _____

Section: _____ Date: _____

Macronutrient Assessment

Sources of Calories

1. Use the "Nutrients Reports" you created in Activity 7.2 to complete the following table. Compare your average daily intake of macronutrients to the Acceptable Macronutrient Distribution Ranges (AMDRs) for a particular calorie source. The AMDR is associated with reduced risk of chronic disease and provides intakes of essential nutrients. An intake outside of the AMDR carries the potential of increased risk for chronic diseases and/or insufficient intake of essential nutrients.

	Average Daily Intake (grams)	Average Kcal from Macronutrient	Average Total Calories*	Share of Total Calories (%)	Recommended Range of Calories (%)
Protein	_____ × 4 =	_____ ÷	_____ =	_____	10–35%
Total Fat	_____ × 9 =	_____ ÷	_____ =	_____	20–35%
Carbohydrates	_____ × 4 =	_____ ÷	_____ =	_____	45–65%

* The "average total calories" should be the same number in each calculation; equal to the average number of calories you eat in one day.

2. Assess how well you met this recommendation for distribution of calories, allowing for no more than a small contribution of calories (less than 10 percent) from alcohol. Do you need to eat more of one macronutrient and less of another to fit within the acceptable ranges?

_____

_____

Protein Intake

1. Was your average percentage of calories from protein 10–35 percent?

_____yes _____no _____ percent calories from protein

2. Your personal recommended dietary allowance (RDA) for protein is based on your healthy weight. Calculate your RDA for protein by following these steps:

   a. Convert your *healthy weight* *in pounds to kilograms (kg): Divide healthy weight in pounds by 2.2 = _____kg

   b. Multiply your healthy weight in kilograms by 0.8 protein/kg weight to determine your RDA for protein: _____kg body weight × 0.8g/kg = _____ g protein.

   *If you are not sure if you are within a healthy weight range, look at the body mass index (BMI) chart found in Chapter 8 (Table 8.2) of *Physical Activity & Health, Fourth Edition.*

3. Did your average protein intake meet or exceed your RDA for protein?

   _____yes _____no

Total Fat Intake

1. Did 20–35 percent of your total calories come from fat?

   _____yes _____no   _____ percent calories from fat

2. Determine your average percentage of total calories from saturated fat:

   Average daily intake of saturated fat = _____ grams

   Multiply by 9 calories/gram = _____ calories from saturated fat

   Divide by your total average calories and multiply by 100 to get percentage of calories from saturated fat.

   Did you meet the *Dietary Guidelines* recommendation of less than 10 percent of your total calories coming from saturated fat?

   _____yes _____no   _____ percent calories from saturated fat

3. Determine your grams from trans fat. Check the nutrition facts label for trans fat content. Also you must check the package labels or ingredients list to see if "partially hydrogenated," "shortening," or "margarine" are listed. If listed, the product most likely contains trans fat. This is because the Food and Drug Administration (FDA) allows food companies to list the amount of trans fat as "0 grams" on the Nutrition Facts panel if the amount of trans fat is less than 0.5 grams per serving.

   Did you meet the *Dietary Guidelines* recommendation of less than 2 grams of trans fat per day?

   _____yes _____no   _____ grams trans fat

   Did you consume any product that had "0 grams" of trans fat listed on the label, but had "partially hydrogenated," "shortening," or "margarine" listed in the ingredients or package label?

   _____

   _____

4. Did you meet the *Dietary Guidelines* recommendation of less than 300 milligrams (mg) of cholesterol per day?

_____yes _____no   _____ mg cholesterol

Total Carbohydrate Intake

1. Did 45–65 percent of your total calories come from carbohydrates?

   _____yes _____no   _____ percent calories from carbohydrates

2. Did you meet the *Dietary Guidelines* recommendation of making half of your grains whole?

   _____yes _____no

3. Did you meet the *Dietary Guidelines* recommendation of varying your veggies? (Vegetables are organized into five subgroups based on their nutrient content: dark green, starchy, red and orange, beans and peas, and other vegetables.)

   _____yes _____no

4. Did you meet the *Dietary Guidelines* recommendation of focusing on fruit? (Any fruit or 100 percent fruit juice counts.)

   _____yes _____no

5. Did you limit added sugars (e.g., high-fructose corn syrup, white sugar, brown sugar, corn syrup, corn syrup solids, raw sugar, maple syrup, fructose sweetener, and honey) to less than 10 percent of your calories?

   _____yes _____no

6. Did you meet the *Dietary Guidelines* recommendation for fiber?

   _____yes _____no   _____ grams of fiber

Describe how well your diet meets the recommendations for macronutrient intake. Compose a short paragraph (five to six sentences) that describes the overall contribution of calories from protein, fat, and carbohydrate in your diet and whether your intake of specific types of protein, fat, and carbohydrate is healthy or excessive.

_____

_____

_____

_____

_____

_____

Name: _____ Course Number: _____

Section: _____ Date: _____

Healthy Eating Behaviors Assessment

The following 13 descriptions of healthy eating behaviors are based on the 2010 *Dietary Guidelines for Americans* recommendations regarding foods and nutrients all Americans should increase or reduce.

Part I. For each statement, check the column that best describes you. Please answer each statement as you currently are (rather than how you think you should be).

2010 Dietary Guideline Recommendations	Never or Rarely	Sometimes	Usually or Always
1. I eat a variety of vegetables, especially dark-green and red and orange vegetables and beans and peas.			
2. I consume at least half of all grains as whole grains and/or increase whole-grain intake by replacing refined grains with whole grains.			
3. I consume fat-free or low-fat milk and milk products, such as milk, yogurt, cheese, or fortified soy beverages.			
4. I choose a variety of protein foods, which include seafood, lean meat and poultry, eggs, beans and peas, soy products, and unsalted nuts and seeds.			
5. I increase the amount and variety of seafood consumed by choosing seafood in place of some meat and poultry.			
6. I replace protein foods that are higher in solid fats with choices that are lower in solid fats and calories, and/or are sources of oils. The fats in meat, poultry, and eggs are considered solid fats, while the fats in seafood, nuts, and seeds are considered oils. Meat and poultry should be consumed in lean forms to decrease intake of solid fats.			
7. I use oils to replace solid fats where possible.			

2010 Dietary Guideline Recommendations	Never or Rarely	Sometimes	Usually or Always
8. I choose foods that provide more potassium, dietary fiber, calcium, and vitamin D, which are nutrients of concern in American diets. These foods include vegetables, fruits, whole grains, and milk and milk products.			
9. I choose and prepare foods with little salt and consume less than 2300 milligrams (mg) of sodium per day.			
10. I consume less than 10 percent of calories from saturated fatty acids by replacing them with monounsaturated and polyunsaturated fatty acids.			
11. I keep trans fatty acid consumption as low as possible by limiting foods that contain synthetic sources of trans fats, such as partially hydrogenated oils, and by limiting other solid fats.			
12. I limit the consumption of foods that contain refined grains, especially refined-grain foods that contain solid fats, added sugars, and sodium.			
13. If I consume alcohol, I consume it in moderation—up to one drink per day for women and two drinks per day for men—and only if I am of legal drinking age.			
Totals			

Source: Data from *Dietary Guidelines for Americans.* (2010). Online http://health.gov/dietaryguidelines/2010.asp.

Part II. Select one behavior that you checked "never or rarely" or "sometimes" that you plan to work on in the next 30 days to begin eating healthier.

Target behavior: _____

Step 1: Your goal is to commit to this target behavior soon. You will do so by setting small, realistic goals and creating a plan to take action.

What changes will you need to make to achieve this target behavior? In other words, what will you need to do differently to succeed?

_____

_____

Write one or two SMART goals that will help you achieve this target behavior:

1. _____

2. _____

Healthy Eating Behaviors Assessment

Commit to take action. Set a start date: _____

Tell someone what you plan to do. Being accountable to others motivates you and also offers you support and encouragement.

Who did you tell? _____

Signature: _____

Step 2: Your goal is to firmly establish this behavior as a lifelong habit by anticipating problems and preparing to overcome failures, and by rewarding your success to stay committed.

Track your progress. For 7 days after your start date, keep track of the results of trying to meet your SMART goal(s) on the following chart:

SMART Goals	Dates	Results

Evaluate your progress and continue or modify your plan:

_____

_____

In what ways have you benefited from adopting this behavior?

_____

_____

What motivates you the most to continue practicing this behavior and why?

_____

_____

Reward your progress. Permanently changing lifestyle behaviors takes patience and consistent positive reinforcement. List several rewards you could give yourself for meeting your goals:

_____

_____

Select a reward for meeting your goal(s) for 7 days: _____

Select a reward for meeting your goal(s) for 1 month: _____

Chapter 7: Critical Thinking Questions

Optimal Nutrition for an Active Lifestyle

1. Like Mare, you might sometimes rely on dietary supplements. What supplements are you currently taking or have you taken? For each supplement, list natural foods that you could eat that provide you the same nutritional value as the supplement.

2. Identify three barriers you face in trying to follow the *Dietary Guidelines for Americans*. For each barrier, identify a strategy and timeline to overcome it.

3. You are one of 12 students at your university who is asked to assist the dietetics staff in developing healthy, nutritious, and appealing meals for college students. Using your nutrition knowledge, develop a well-balanced menu for breakfast, lunch, and dinner.

4. Go to a local health food store (often you can find one in a shopping mall). Walk through the store and look at the products and their health claims. Find two products, identify the claims made, and note any scientific research that supports the claim. Would you, based on the information provided, use this product? Why or why not?

——

——

——

——

——

——

——

——

——

——

——

——

——

——

Critical Thinking Questions

Name: _____ Course Number: _____

Section: _____ Date: _____

Assessing Your Weight and Health Risk

Assessment of weight and health risk involves using three key measures: body mass index, waist circumference, and risk factors for diseases and conditions associated with obesity.

Step 1: Body Mass Index (BMI) Measurement

BMI measures your weight in relation to your height. It is used to identify people at risk for some health problems. Higher BMI values indicate greater weight per unit of height. BMI is considered a more accurate measurement of body fat than weight alone in people 20 years of age or older. For assessment of young people ages 2 to 20 years, use Appendix B: Growth Charts: Stature-for-Age and Weight-for-Age Percentiles for Children and Teenagers in *Physical Activity & Health, Fourth Edition*.

Calculate your BMI using the formula: $BMI = \dfrac{\text{weight (pounds)} \times 703}{\text{height squared (inches}^2)}$

For example, for someone who is 5 feet, 7 inches tall (e.g., 67 inches) and weighs 190 pounds, the calculation looks like this:

$$BMI = \frac{192 \times 703}{67 \times 67} = \frac{134{,}976}{4489} = 30.07$$

Your height in inches _____   Calculate your BMI:

Your weight in pounds _____

Using your height and weight compare your calculated BMI to the BMI values in the text. They should be the same.

Are you at increased risk due to BMI? _____ yes _____ no (Refer to the following table.)

Body Mass Index	Category	Health Risks
<18.5	Underweight	No risks unless waist circumference indicates risk
18.5–24.9	Healthy weight	No risks unless waist circumference indicates risk
25.0–29.9	Overweight	Moderate risk
≥ 30.0	Obese	High risk

Although BMI is a useful measure for predicting health risks associated with excess weight due to fat, it does have limitations. It may overestimate body fat in lean, muscular athletes and underestimate body fat in older persons and others who have lost muscle. In addition, BMI provides no information about fat distribution (site of fat), which is an important risk factor in obesity-related health problems.

Step 2: Waist Circumference Measurement

Where you carry your weight affects your risk for a variety of health problems. If fat tends to gather in your abdominal area, you may have increased health risks. No matter what your height or build, an increased waistline is a sign that you could be at greater risk for developing serious ongoing health problems. Waist measurement is often seen as a better way of checking a person's risk for developing a number of health problems from obesity than BMI. Recording changes over time in waist circumference is important because it can change even when body weight stays the same.

Directions: To measure your waist circumference, place a tape measure or a piece of string around your bare abdomen just above the hip bones (see diagram). Pull the tape or string so it is snug, but not compressing the skin, and is parallel to the floor. Relax your abdominal muscles (not pulled in), exhale normally, and measure your waist. If you use a piece of string, use a yardstick or other measuring device to measure the string.

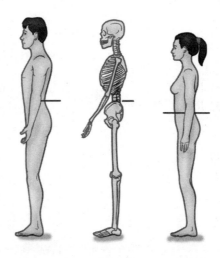

Measuring-Tape Position for Waist Circumference in Adults.

Record your waist circumference _____ inches.

Are you at increased risk due to waist circumference? _____ yes _____ no
(Refer to the following table.)

Assessing Your Weight and Health Risk

Waist Measurement Classification Table		
Health Risks	**Women**	**Men**
Low risk	<32 inches (80 cm)	<37 inches (94 cm)
Moderate risk	32–35 inches (80–88 cm)	37–40 inches (94–102 cm)
High risk	>35 inches (88 cm)	>40 inches (102 cm)

Step 3: Risk Factors and Conditions to Consider if Overweight or Obese

If you are classified as overweight or obese based on your BMI and waist circumference measures, there are associated risk factors and conditions that need to be assessed. Do you have any of the following risk factors or conditions?

Risk Factors to Consider if Overweight or Obese	Yes	No
High blood pressure (hypertension)		
High low-density lipoprotein (LDL) cholesterol		
Low high-density lipoprotein (HDL) cholesterol		
High triglycerides		
High blood glucose		
Family history of premature heart disease		
Physical inactivity		
Cigarette smoking		
Conditions to Consider if Overweight or Obese		
Established coronary heart disease		
Presence of other atherosclerotic diseases (e.g., peripheral artery disease, symptomatic carotid artery disease)		
Type 2 diabetes		
Sleep apnea		
Osteoarthritis		

Step 4: Overall Assessment and Subsequent Decisions Based on BMI, Waist Circumference, and Associated Health Risks and Conditions.

- If your BMI is between 25 and 30 and you are otherwise healthy, try to avoid gaining more weight, and look into healthy ways to lose weight and increase physical activity. Plan on setting a weight-loss goal if:

    ○ Your BMI is 30 or above, *or*

    ○ Your BMI is between 25 and 30 *and* you have:

        ▪ Two or more risk factors or conditions *or*

        ▪ A family history of heart disease or diabetes, *or*

    ○ Your waist measures over 40 inches (men) or 35 inches (women)—even if your BMI is less than 25—and you have:

        ▪ Two or more risk factors or conditions *or*

        ▪ A family history of heart disease or diabetes.

If you have a BMI or a waist circumference measure, or risks that put you at higher risk for health problems, don't despair. The good news is even a small weight loss (between 5 and 10 percent of your current weight) will provide many health benefits and help lower your risk of developing many chronic health problems.

Step 5: Setting a Weight-Loss Goal

If you are at risk for a weight-related health problem you need to begin thinking about setting a weight-loss goal. Goal setting motivates us to achieve. As you plan your weight-loss goal, keep in mind that slow is the way to go. Losing too much weight to quickly can be unsafe. Keep in mind that you are setting a short-term goal. Setting and achieving several short-term goals will ultimately allow you to attain your long-term weight-loss goal.

Use one of the following three methods to set your weight-loss goal. The method you choose will likely depend on your current weight and your personal preferences.

1. **Lose 5 percent of weight over 3 months.** The National Heart, Lung, and Blood Institute and the North American Association for the Study of Obesity recommend an initial weight-loss goal of 5 percent of your current weight over a 3-month period. For example, someone weighing 180 pounds should not plan on losing more than 9 pounds over a 3-month period. Even if you have more weight to lose, aiming for a 5-percent loss will keep you focused on a short-term achievable target and heighten your chances of maintaining this loss long term. After you lose 5 percent successfully, you can set a new short-term goal. To determine how many pounds equal 5 percent of your weight, do these calculations:

Your current weight in pounds _____ × 0.05 = _____ pounds to lose.

Current weight _____ minus _____ pounds to lose = _____ my new 3-month weight goal.

2. Lose .5 to 2 pounds per week. No matter what your goal weight, the healthiest and most long-lasting fat loss typically occurs in weekly increments of .5 to 2 pounds. Losing weight more rapidly than this results in the majority of weight lost being water and muscle rather than fat. Someone who is very overweight can aim for a weekly weight loss at the higher end of the weekly range, while those who are only slightly overweight should aim for the middle or lower end.

3. Use the BMI or waist circumference charts. Estimate a weight that you think will put you in the healthy weight or waist range.

Considering your current BMI, waist circumference, and the risks associated with being overweight or obese, what do you consider a safe weight change goal for you?

Weight change goal: _____ maintain weight in current range

_____ lose pounds _____ by _____

_____ gain pounds _____ by _____

Waist circumference goal: _____ maintain waist circumference in current range

_____ lose inches _____ by _____

Whether you want to maintain, lose, or gain weight depends on your energy balance. Energy is another word for "calories." What you eat and drink is energy in; what you burn through physical activity is energy out. The *Physical Activity Guidelines for Americans* recommend at least 30 minutes of moderate-intensity activity on most days of the week to obtain health benefits and reduce the risk of chronic disease. You can gain greater health benefits from doing more activity. To help manage your body weight and prevent gradual weight gain, 60 minutes of moderate to vigorous activity on most days of the week may be necessary. For both weight maintenance and weight loss, it is important to keep food and drink intake (calories) at a level that is equal to or less than the amount of calories you burn through daily activity. You can determine your energy balance by completing Activity 8.2.

Name: ———————————————————————— Course Number: ————————————————

Section: ———————————————————————— Date: ————————————————

Determining Your Energy Balance

Directions: Calculate your total daily energy expenditure using the following formula and steps.

Total Energy Expenditure = Resting Metabolic Rate (RMR) × Physical Activity Multiplier

Step 1: Calculate your RMR.*

Female RMR:

RMR = −161 + 10(weight in pounds ÷ 2.2) + 6.25(height in inches × 2.54) − 5 (age)

RMR = −161 + 10(_____ ÷ 2.2) + 6.25(_____ × 2.54) − 5 (age)

Male RMR:

RMR = 5 + 10(weight in pounds ÷ 2.2) + 6.25(height in inches × 2.54) − 5 (age)

RMR = −161 + 10(_____ ÷ 2.2) + 6.25(_____ × 2.54) − 5 (age)

My RMR is _____.

Example:

Sex: Female   Height: 5 foot, 7 inches (e.g., 67 inches)

Age: 35   Weight: 206 pounds

RMR = −161 + 10(206 ÷ 2.2) + 6.25(67 × 2.54) − 5 (35)

RMR = −161 + 936 + 1064 − 175

RMR = 1664

Note: The Mifflin–St Jeor equation employed in Step 1 to calculate RMR is available as an interactive calculator online at http://www.calculator.net/calorie-calculator.html.

* *Source:* Reproduced with permission from Mifflin, MD, St Jeor, ST, Hill, LA, Scott, BJ, Daugerty, SA, & Koh, YO. (1990). A new predictive equation for resting energy expenditure in healthy individuals. *American Journal of Clinical Nutrition* (1990; 51: 241–247).

Step 2: Assess your physical activity level and calculate your physical activity multiplier.

Sedentary (little or no exercise, desk job) = RMR × 1.2

Light activity (light exercise/sports 1–3 days per week) = RMR × 1.375

Moderately active (moderate exercise/sports 3–5 days per week) = RMR × 1.5

Very active (hard exercise/sports 6–7 days per week) = RMR × 1.75

Extremely active (hard daily exercise/sports and physical job) = RMR × 1.9

My physical activity multiplier is _____.

Step 3: Calculate total daily energy expenditure by multiplying RMR by the appropriate physical activity multiplier.

RMR _____ × Physical Activity Multiplier _____ = Total Daily Energy Expenditure

My total daily energy expenditure is _____ calories.

Example from Step 1:

Sex: Female	Height: 5 foot, 7 inches	Activity level: light
Age: 35	Weight: 206 pounds	
RMR = 1664		
1664 × 1.375 = 2288		

Note: The physical activity multipliers by physical activity level employed in Step 2 are available as an interactive calculator online at http://www.calculator.net/calorie-calculator.html.

Based on these calculations, this woman's daily calorie needs are 2288. This is an estimate of the number of calories she needs to consume each day to maintain her weight at 206 pounds. If she consumes less and maintains her activity level, she will lose weight. If she eats more than 2288 calories and maintains her activity level, she will gain weight.

Step 4: Compare your daily caloric intake with your daily caloric expenditure.

Use the "Nutrients Reports" you completed for Activity 7.2 based on your daily diet records with your daily energy expenditure (complete for a week):

Day 1:   Intake was _____ kcal   Expenditure was _____ kcal

Day 2:   Intake was _____ kcal   Expenditure was _____ kcal

Day 3:   Intake was _____ kcal   Expenditure was _____ kcal

Day 4:   Intake was _____ kcal   Expenditure was _____ kcal

Day 5:   Intake was _____ kcal   Expenditure was _____ kcal

Day 6:   Intake was _____ kcal   Expenditure was _____ kcal

Day 7:   Intake was _____ kcal   Expenditure was _____ kcal

Step 5: Compare your average energy intake with your average energy expenditure. Divide your total intake values and your total expenditure values listed by the number of days.

Average intake of calories per day: _____ kcal/day

Average expenditure of calories per day: _____ kcal/day

Step 6: What is the average difference? _____ kcal/day

What is the direction of the difference?

_____ Intake sometimes greater, expenditure sometimes greater; balances out over time.

_____ Intake more often greater than expenditure.

_____ Expenditure greater than intake.

Step 7: Is this difference a true reflection of your tendency to gain, lose, or maintain weight?

_____ yes _____ no

If not, explain why:

(Possible explanations include underreporting intake, overreporting energy expenditure, and days not typical. Ideally, your recorded days will be typical.)

_____

_____

_____

Step 8: Unbalancing the energy balance for weight loss.

One pound of body fat is equal to 3500 calories. The best way to create a negative energy balance is through a combination of reduced caloric intake and increased caloric expenditure. The recommended amount of fat loss in a week is 1 pound. This is best accomplished by creating a 3500 weekly calorie deficit or 500 daily calorie deficit. Lowering your caloric intake (dietary modification) or increasing energy expenditure (physical activity modification) can be effective independently in obtaining the recommended 3500 weekly calorie deficit, but a combination of both produces the best results. In other words, reducing daily caloric expenditure by 250 calories and increasing physical activity by 250 calories will produce the best results. Increasing the weekly energy deficit above 3500 calories could cause a significant loss of water and muscle and be counterproductive to your goal of losing body fat.

Based on your weight loss goal from Activity 8.1:

What are some ways to increase your daily energy expenditure by 250 calories?

_____

_____

_____

What are some ways to decrease your daily energy intake by 250 calories?

_____

_____

_____

Name: ———————————— Course Number: ————————————

Section: ———————————— Date: ————————————

Tracking Your Weight and Health Risk

Test 1 Date: ————————

Measurement	Value	Exceeds Standard Yes or No
BMI		
Waist circumference		
Risk factor ————————		
Risk factor ————————		
Risk factor ————————		

Test 2 Date: ————————

Measurement	Value	Exceeds Standard Yes or No
BMI		
Waist circumference		
Risk factor ————————		
Risk factor ————————		
Risk factor ————————		

Test 3 Date: ————————

Measurement	Value	Exceeds Standard Yes or No
BMI		
Waist circumference		
Risk factor ————————		
Risk factor ————————		
Risk factor ————————		

Test 4 Date: _____

Measurement	Value	Exceeds Standard Yes or No
BMI		
Waist circumference		
Risk factor _____		
Risk factor _____		
Risk factor _____		

Test 5 Date: _____

Measurement	Value	Exceeds Standard Yes or No
BMI		
Waist circumference		
Risk factor _____		
Risk factor _____		
Risk factor _____		

Test 6 Date: _____

Measurement	Value	Exceeds Standard Yes or No
BMI		
Waist circumference		
Risk factor _____		
Risk factor _____		
Risk factor _____		

Test 7 Date: _____

Measurement	Value	Exceeds Standard Yes or No
BMI		
Waist circumference		
Risk factor _____		
Risk factor _____		
Risk factor _____		

Tracking Your Weight and Health Risk

Name: _____ Course Number: _____

Section: _____ Date: _____

How Do You Feel About Your Body?

	Quite Satisfied	Somewhat Satisfied	Somewhat Dissatisfied	Very Dissatisfied
Hair	_____	_____	_____	_____
Arms	_____	_____	_____	_____
Hands	_____	_____	_____	_____
Feet	_____	_____	_____	_____
Waist	_____	_____	_____	_____
Buttocks	_____	_____	_____	_____
Hips	_____	_____	_____	_____
Legs and ankles	_____	_____	_____	_____
Thighs	_____	_____	_____	_____
Chest or breasts	_____	_____	_____	_____
Posture	_____	_____	_____	_____
General attractiveness	_____	_____	_____	_____

1. Which of your thoughts and actions enhance your body image?

_____

_____

2. Which of your thoughts and actions are detrimental to your body image?

_____

_____

3. What societal forces (e.g., expectations of friends and parents, advertising, celebrities and professional athletes) influence your body image most strongly?

_____

_____

4. How susceptible are you to media images of "ideal" body proportions for members of your sex?

_____

_____

5. What could you do to become more satisfied with your body image?

_____

_____

Source: Reproduced from G. Edlin & E. Golanty. (2007). *For Your Health: A Study Guide and Self-Assessment Workbook.* Sudbury, MA: Jones & Bartlett, 77.

Name: _____ Course Number: _____

Section: _____ Date: _____

Chapter 8: Critical Thinking Questions

Achieving and Maintaining a Healthy Weight

1. From the vignette, how would you assess Leah's preoccupation with her weight? What factors influence her concerns about her weight? Do you believe she has an unhealthy obsession with her weight?

2. On your campus, identify and briefly describe the resources available for students regarding healthy weight management and eating disorders.

3. Your housemate, Linda, goes on a new fad diet that was recently reported by a respected national morning TV show. Linda reports that this new diet will allow her to lose 10 pounds by Saturday (6 days from now). Explain to Linda why this fad diet will not work, and if she were to lose the 10 pounds in 6 days, what would likely happen.

4. As a residence hall assistant (RA) you have been asked by your floor to talk about obesity and how as college freshmen they can manage their weight sensibly. In your talk, discuss healthy weight, overweight and obesity, body mass index, and the importance of good nutrition and physical activity.

_____

_____

_____

_____

_____

_____

_____

_____

_____

_____

_____

_____

_____

_____

Critical Thinking Questions

Name: _____ Course Number: _____

Section: _____ Date: _____

Are You Consuming Enough Calcium?

According to statistics from the U.S. Department of Agriculture, only 1 in 10 girls and 1 in 3 boys ages 12 to 19 in the United States get the Recommended Dietary Allowance (RDA) of calcium, placing them at serious risk for osteoporosis and other bone diseases. Because nearly 90 percent of adult bone mass is established by the end of this age range, the nation's young adults stand in the midst of a calcium deficiency crisis. The daily calcium requirements by age and sex is listed below.

Age and Sex	Adequate Daily Intake of Calcium (mg)
Infants, male or female, 0–6 months	210
Infants, male or female, 7–12 months	270
Children, male or female, 1–3 years	500
Children, male or female, 4–8 years	800
Males and females, 9–18 years	1300
Males and females,* 19–50	1000
Males and females,† 51 years and older	1200
Pregnant or lactating female, 14–18 years	1300
Pregnant or lactating female, 19–50 years	1000

*If you are female and in menopause, you should increase your calcium intake to 1200 mg.

†Some clinicians recommend 1500 mg of calcium per day for postmenopausal women.

Source: Reproduced from I.M. Alexander. (2006). 100 Questions and Answers About Osteoporosis and Osteopenia. Sudbury, MA: Jones & Bartlett, 95.

Record your calcium intake from the foods you eat for a week (see Table 9.2 in your textbook for a list of selected food sources of calcium). Are you obtaining enough calcium in your diet from food? If not, what foods could you include in your diet to increase your daily calcium intake?

_____

_____

Have you thought about taking a dietary calcium supplement? Why or why not?

_____

_____

Name: ——————————————————————— Course Number: ———————————

Section: ——————————————————————— Date: ———————————————

Are You Performing Enough Weight-Bearing Exercise?

Physical activity plays an important role in improving bone health, specifically because bone mass is responsive to mechanical loads (stress) placed on the skeleton. Bone becomes stronger and denser when you place demands on it. Examples of weight-bearing exercises for adults are listed here.

Weight-Bearing Exercise for Adults

The best exercise for your bones is weight-bearing activities, which cause muscles and bones to work against gravity. Some examples of weight-bearing exercises include:

- Brisk walking
- Hiking
- Stair climbing
- Jumping rope
- Jogging or running
- Dancing
- Downhill skiing
- Golf (which includes shouldering the golf bag around for 18 holes)

- Yoga (performing the slow, precise Iyengar style or the vigorous ashtanga)
- Weight lifting or resistance training
- Tennis or racquetball
- Field hockey
- Basketball
- Volleyball
- Soccer
- Lacrosse

Note: Take a few exercise precautions if you already have low bone mass, osteopenia, or osteoporosis because your fracture risk is higher than normal. Be cautious about trying any exercise with the potential for serious falls, like downhill skiing, and check with your healthcare provider before starting any new exercise program, especially if you're taking medications that slow your coordination or throw off your balance.

Source: Adapted from Centers for Disease Control and Prevention. (2013). Weight-Bearing Physical Activity. Online: http://www.cdc.gov/nutrition/everyone/basics/vitamins/ calcium.html; and the National Institute of Arthritis and Musculoskeletal and Skin Diseases (NIAMS). (2013). Exercise for Your Bone Health. Online: http://www.niams.nih.gov/health_info/bone/bone_health/exercise/default.asp.

Which of the weight-bearing exercises listed above do you regularly perform on a daily or weekly basis?

———

———

———

———

Based on the scientific information provided in Chapter 9 on the role of physical activity and bone health, do you feel that your current physical activity program related to weight-bearing and resistance exercises is adequate for your skeletal health? Why or why not?

_____

_____

_____

_____

_____

_____

_____

_____

_____

_____

_____

_____

_____

_____

_____

_____

_____

_____

_____

_____

_____

_____

_____

_____

_____

Are You Performing Enough Weight-Bearing Exercise?

Name: _____ Course Number: _____

Section: _____ Date: _____

My Osteoporosis Risk

Directions

1. Go to the online assessment tool "Your Disease Risk: The Source on Prevention" at http://www.yourdiseaserisk.wustl.edu. Here, you can find out your risk of developing osteoporosis in the United States and get personalized tips for preventing osteoporosis.

2. Click the What's your osteoporosis risk? link, and then click Questionnaire.

3. Is your risk low, average, or high? _____

4. Click the What makes up my risk? button and list the factors that raise your risk and the factors that lower your risk.

Factors that raise my risk of osteoporosis: _____

Factors that lower my risk of osteoporosis: _____

Chapter 9: Critical Thinking Questions

Achieving Optimal Bone Health

1. Like Julie, many people do not understand that both physical inactivity and low calcium intake are key factors in the development of osteoporosis. You have been asked by a local ninth-grade health teacher to explain to her students the importance of physical activity and nutrition in preventing osteoporosis (a condition that is the last thing on most ninth-graders' minds). In 250 words or less, explain their importance.

2. Review the factors that affect osteoporosis (genetic, hormonal, nutritional, and lifestyle). Review your family history to determine if you are at risk of osteoporosis. Then select two other factors and, based on your current behaviors, decide what behaviors you could change that would assist in preventing osteoporosis. List them.

3. "Physical activity and nutrition are key elements in achieving optimal bone density during the first 20 to 30 years of life and maintaining bone density throughout life." Provide information that supports this statement.

_____

_____

_____

_____

_____

_____

_____

_____

_____

_____

_____

_____

_____

_____

_____

Name: _____ Course Number: _____

Section: _____ Date: _____

Determining Your Mental Stress Balance

The "hassles and uplifts" theory of stress maintains that at the end of each day we create a mental balance sheet. If the daily hassles outweigh the daily uplifts, we've had a bad day. If the uplifts outweigh the hassles, we've had a good day. Hassles are the irritating, frustrating, distressing demands of everyday life that grind us down. By contrast, uplifts are the positive experiences that bring us joy and pleasure that tend to "make our day."

Negative Event Scale

You are asked to think about the negative events (hassles) that you have *experienced in the last month*. Negative daily events are the small day-to-day happenings that lead people to feel hassled. From such events people can feel distressed, upset, guilty, or scared. Negative events can also lead to people feeling hostile, irritable, nervous, afraid, ashamed, or frustrated.

Following are a list of 57 items that can be negative events. For each item, consider first, if the event occurred *during the last month* and then how **hassled** you felt. Circle 0 if it did not occur, 1 if the event occurred but you did not experience any hassle, 2 if it occurred and was a little of a hassle, 3 if it occurred and was somewhat of a hassle, 4 if it occurred and was a lot of a hassle, and 5 if the event occurred and was an extreme hassle.

Please remember that it is important that you:
      * circle one number for *each item even if there was no hassle.*
      * consider each item with only *the last month in mind*.

How much of a <u>hassle</u> was this negative event?	0 = Did not occur 1 = Event occurred but there was no hassle 2 = Event occurred and a little of a hassle 3 = Event occurred and somewhat of a hassle 4 = Event occurred and a lot of a hassle
In the last month	5 = Event occurred and an extreme hassle

Problems with Friends

1. Negative feedback from your friend/s	0	1	2	3	4	5
2. Negative communication with friend/s	0	1	2	3	4	5
3. Conflict with a friend/s	0	1	2	3	4	5
4. Disagreement (including arguments) with a friend/s	0	1	2	3	4	5

Problems with your Spouse/Partner (boy/girl friend)

5. Negative communication with your spouse/partner (boy/girl friend)	0	1	2	3	4	5
6. Conflict with spouse/partner (boy/girl friend)	0	1	2	3	4	5
7. Disagreement (including arguments) with spouse/partner (boy/girl friend)	0	1	2	3	4	5
8. Rejection by your spouse/partner (boy/girl friend)	0	1	2	3	4	5
9. Your spouse/partner (boy/girl friend) let you down	0	1	2	3	4	5

Work (if employed)

10. The nature of your job/work	0	1	2	3	4	5
11. Your work load	0	1	2	3	4	5
12. Meeting deadlines or goals on the job	0	1	2	3	4	5
13. Use of your skills at work	0	1	2	3	4	5

Money

14. Not enough money for necessities (e.g., food, clothing, housing, health care, taxes, insurance)	0	1	2	3	4	5
15. Not enough money for education	0	1	2	3	4	5
16. Not enough money for emergencies	0	1	2	3	4	5
17. Not enough money for extras (e.g., entertainment, recreation, vacations)	0	1	2	3	4	5

Problems with Children

18. Negative communication with your child(ren)	0	1	2	3	4	5
19. Conflict with your child(ren)	0	1	2	3	4	5
20. Disagreement (including arguments) with your child(ren)	0	1	2	3	4	5

School

21. Your study load	0	1	2	3	4	5
22. Study/course deadlines	0	1	2	3	4	5
23. Time pressures	0	1	2	3	4	5
24. Problems getting assignments/essays finished	0	1	2	3	4	5

Problems with Teachers/Lecturers

25. Negative communication with teacher/s, lecturer/s	0	1	2	3	4	5
26. Negative feedback from teacher/s, lecturer/s	0	1	2	3	4	5
27. Conflict with teacher/s, lecturer/s	0	1	2	3	4	5
28. Disagreement (including arguments) with your teacher/s, lecturer/s	0	1	2	3	4	5

Problems with Parents or Parents-in-Law

29. Negative communication with your parents or parents-in-law	0	1	2	3	4	5
30. Conflict with your parents or parents-in-law	0	1	2	3	4	5

31. Disagreement (including arguments) with parents   0   1   2   3   4   5
or parents-in-law
32. Negative feedback from your parents or parents-in-law   0   1   2   3   4   5

Problems with Other Students

33. Negative communication with other student/s   0   1   2   3   4   5
34. Conflict with other student/s   0   1   2   3   4   5
35. Disagreement (including arguments) with   0   1   2   3   4   5
other student/s
36. Doing things with other student/s   0   1   2   3   4   5

Problems with Relative(s)

37. Conflict with other relative   0   1   2   3   4   5
38. Disagreement (including arguments) with other relative   0   1   2   3   4   5
39. Negative feedback from other relative   0   1   2   3   4   5
40. Doing things with other relative   0   1   2   3   4   5

Health Problems

41. Your health   0   1   2   3   4   5
42. Your physical abilities   0   1   2   3   4   5
43. Your medical care   0   1   2   3   4   5
44. Getting sick (e.g., flu, colds)   0   1   2   3   4   5

Problems with Your Work Supervisor/Employer

45. Negative feedback from your supervisor/employer   0   1   2   3   4   5
46. Negative communication with your supervisor/employer   0   1   2   3   4   5
47. Conflict with your supervisor/employer   0   1   2   3   4   5
48. Disagreement (including arguments) with your   0   1   2   3   4   5
supervisor/employer

Hassles of Getting a Job

49. Finding a job (e.g., interviews, placements)   0   1   2   3   4   5
50. Finding work   0   1   2   3   4   5
51. Problems with finding a job   0   1   2   3   4   5
52. Employment problems (e.g., finding, losing a job)   0   1   2   3   4   5

Academic Limitations

53. Not getting the marks (results) you expected   0   1   2   3   4   5
54. Your academic ability not as good as you thought   0   1   2   3   4   5
55. Not understanding some subjects   0   1   2   3   4   5

Course Interest   0   1   2   3   4   5

56. Course not relevant to your future career   0   1   2   3   4   5
57. Your course is boring   0   1   2   3   4   5

Source: Courtesy of Darrly Mayberry, PhD, Monash University Department of Rural and Indigenous Health, Melbourne, Australia.

Positive Event Scale

The positive event scale asks you to think about the positive (uplifting) events that you have *experienced in the last month*. Positive daily events are the small day-to-day happenings that lead people to feel uplifted. From such events people can feel inspired, alert, attentive, or active. Positive events can also lead to feeling emotions such as interest, excitement, strength, pride, determination, and enthusiasm.

Following are a list of 41 items that can be positive events. For each item, consider first if the event occurred *during the last month* and second how **uplifted** (i.e., the amount of positive uplifting emotion) it made you feel. Circle 0 if it did not occur, 1 if the event occurred but you did not experience any uplift, 2 if it occurred and was a little uplifting, 3 if it occurred and was somewhat uplifting, 4 if it occurred and was a lot of an uplift, and 5 if the event occurred and was extremely uplifting.

Please remember that it is important that you:
      * circle one number for *each item even if there was no uplift.*
      * consider each item only with *the last month in mind.*

How <u>uplifted</u> did you feel by this positive event?	
	0 = Did not occur
	1 = Event occurred but was no uplift
	2 = Event occurred and a little uplifting
	3 = Event occurred and somewhat uplifting
	4 = Event occurred, a lot uplifting
In the last month	5 = Event occurred and extremely uplifting

Your Friends

1. Support received from friend/s	0 1 2 3 4 5
2. Support given to friend/s	0 1 2 3 4 5
3. Positive feedback from your friend/s	0 1 2 3 4 5
4. Positive communication with friend/s	0 1 2 3 4 5

Work (if employed)

5. The nature of your job/work	0 1 2 3 4 5
6. Your job security	0 1 2 3 4 5
7. Use of your skills in your work	0 1 2 3 4 5
8. The ideas you have at work	0 1 2 3 4 5

Teachers/Lecturers

9. Support received from teacher/s, lecturer/s	0 1 2 3 4 5
10. Support given to teacher/s, lecturer/s	0 1 2 3 4 5
11. Positive communication with teacher/s, lecturer/s	0 1 2 3 4 5
12. Positive feedback from teacher/s, lecturer/s	0 1 2 3 4 5
13. Doing enjoyable things with teacher/s, lecturer/s	0 1 2 3 4 5

Determining Your Mental Stress Balance

Social Events

14. Going to a party	0	1	2	3	4	5
15. Going out for drinks (e.g., friend's place)	0	1	2	3	4	5
16. Going to the pub	0	1	2	3	4	5
17. Recent social events	0	1	2	3	4	5

School

18. Nature of your course/study	0	1	2	3	4	5
19. Your study load	0	1	2	3	4	5
20. Study/course deadlines	0	1	2	3	4	5
21. University (college) life	0	1	2	3	4	5

Relationship with Spouse/Partner (boy/girl friend)

22. Intimate times with someone	0	1	2	3	4	5
23. Doing enjoyable things with your spouse/partner (boy/girl friend)	0	1	2	3	4	5
24. Positive feedback from spouse/partner (girl/boy friend)	0	1	2	3	4	5
25. Positive communication with spouse/partner (girl/boy friend)	0	1	2	3	4	5
26. Support given to spouse/partner (girl/boy friend)	0	1	2	3	4	5
27. Support received from spouse/partner (girl/boy friend)	0	1	2	3	4	5

Parents or Parents-in-Law

28. Positive feedback from your parents or parents-in-law	0	1	2	3	4	5
29. Positive communication with your parents/parents-in-law	0	1	2	3	4	5
30. Good times with your parents/parents-in-law	0	1	2	3	4	5
31. Support given to your parents/parents-in-law	0	1	2	3	4	5
32. Support received from your parents/parents-in-law	0	1	2	3	4	5

Other Students

33. Support received from other student/s	0	1	2	3	4	5
34. Support given to other student/s	0	1	2	3	4	5
35. Positive communication with other student/s	0	1	2	3	4	5
36. Positive feedback from other student/s	0	1	2	3	4	5

Interactions at Work (if employed)

37. Support given to your supervisor/employer	0	1	2	3	4	5
38. Support received from other workers	0	1	2	3	4	5
39. Support given to other workers	0	1	2	3	4	5
40. Positive feedback from other workers	0	1	2	3	4	5
41. Doing enjoyable things with other workers	0	1	2	3	4	5

Source: Courtesy of Darrly Mayberry, PhD, Monash University Department of Rural and Indigenous Health, Melbourne, Australia.

Any negative events for which you scored a 4 or 5 are considered chronic stressors. How can you modify your perceptions of these stressors and reduce the amount of hassle you feel?

_____

_____

_____

_____

The "hassles and uplifts" theory of stress maintains that we can take control and turn stressful days around by recognizing and creating more uplifts for ourselves. What are some ways to increase your daily uplifts or positive experiences?

_____

_____

_____

_____

Scientists are finding that an attitude of gratitude is a powerful contributor to a happier life. A good way to cultivate gratitude is to keep a journal of good things that happen to you every day. To get started, list 5 things that "**Went Right Today**" for you.

1. _____

2. _____

3. _____

4. _____

5. _____

Name: _____ Course Number: _____

Section: _____ Date: _____

K6 Serious Psychological Distress Assessment

Answer the following questions by checking the box that best applies.

During the past 30 days, how often did you feel . . .	All of the time 4	Most of the time 3	Some of the time 2	A little of the time 1	None of the time 0
So sad that nothing could cheer you up?					
Nervous?					
Restless or fidgety?					
Hopeless?					
That everything was an effort?					
Worthless?					
Total					

Scoring: To score the K6, add the points for each of the questions together. Scores can range from 0 to 24. A threshold of 13 or more points indicates a high degree of distress and possibility of serious mental illness.

Source: Reproduced from National Center for Health Statistics. (2007). Serious psychological distress. Online: http://www.cdc.gov/nchs/data/ad/ad382.pdf.

Name: _____ Course Number: _____

Section: _____ Date: _____

Time Management

Activity 1: Ranking Tasks

Step 1

Write down all the things you need to get done today with no regard to order of importance.

1. _____ 6. _____

2. _____ 7. _____

3. _____ 8. _____

4. _____ 9. _____

5. _____ 10. _____

Step 2

In column A, list all the things that must get done as soon as possible. In column C, list all the things you would like to do, but that are not essential. In column B, put everything else.

A	B	C
_____	_____	_____
_____	_____	_____
_____	_____	_____
_____	_____	_____

Activity 2: Scheduling

After completing Activity 1, complete your schedule.

7:00 a.m. _____

7:30 a.m. _____

8:00 a.m. _____

8:30 a.m. _____

9:00 a.m. _____

9:30 a.m. _____

10:00 a.m. _____

10:30 a.m. _____

11:00 a.m. _____

11:30 a.m. _____

12:00 p.m. _____

12:30 p.m. _____

1:00 p.m. _____

1:30 p.m. _____

2:00 p.m. _____

2:30 p.m. _____

3:00 p.m. _____

3:30 p.m. _____

4:00 p.m. _____

4:30 p.m. _____

5:00 p.m. _____

5:30 p.m. _____

6:00 p.m. _____

6:30 p.m. _____

7:00 p.m. _____

7:30 p.m. _____

8:00 p.m. _____

8:30 p.m. _____

9:00 p.m. _____

9:30 p.m. _____

10:00 p.m. _____

10:30 p.m. _____

11:00 p.m. _____

Name: _____ Course Number: _____

Section: _____ Date: _____

Relaxation Techniques

Activity 1: Progressive Muscle Relaxation

Progressive muscle relaxation involves three steps that can help you actually feel the difference between tension and relaxation. First, tense a muscle and notice how it feels. Second, release the tension and pay attention to that feeling. Third, rest, concentrating on the difference between the two sensations. Perform these steps while either sitting or lying down, preferably in a quiet, soothing environment.

It takes only about 10 minutes to exercise all the major muscle groups. There are several sequences. You can start with the hand muscles, progressing to others; begin at the top, moving from head to toe; or reverse the direction, going from bottom to top as explained in the following section.

Procedure

This sequence of exercises progresses from the feet to the head and takes about 10 minutes. Its effectiveness comes from alternately tensing and relaxing each muscle group. Hold tense, then relax for about 5 seconds each.

1. Curl toes tightly. Hold, Relax, Rest
2. Flex the feet. Hold, Relax, Rest
3. Tighten the calves. Hold, Relax, Rest
4. Tense the thighs. Hold, Relax, Rest
5. Tighten the buttocks. Hold, Relax, Rest
6. Tighten the lower back. Hold, Relax, Rest
7. Tighten the abdomen. Hold, Relax, Rest
8. Tense the upper chest. Hold, Relax, Rest
9. Tense the upper back muscles. Hold, Relax, Rest
10. Clench the fists. Hold, Relax, Rest
11. Extend the fingers and flex the wrists. Hold, Relax, Rest
12. Tighten the forearms. Hold, Relax, Rest
13. Tighten the upper arms. Hold, Relax, Rest
14. Lift the shoulders gently toward the ears. Hold, Relax, Rest

15. Wrinkle the forehead. Hold, Relax, Rest

16. Squeeze your eyes shut. Hold, Relax, Rest

17. Drop your chin, letting your mouth open wide. Hold, Relax, Rest

18. Lift the shoulders gently and then pull them down as if you had weights in the hands. Hold, Relax, Rest

Activity 2: The Relaxation Response

The relaxation response tends to banish inner stress and exert a calming, healing influence. It not only helps preserve emotional balance in everyday life, but it also enhances therapy for a host of illnesses, especially high blood pressure. Herbert Benson developed the following simple, practical procedure for eliciting the relaxation response.

Procedure

1. Select a focus word or brief phrase that has deep meaning for you.

2. Take a comfortable sitting position in a quiet environment.

3. Close your eyes and consciously relax your muscles.

4. Breathe slowly and naturally through your nose while silently repeating your focus word or phrase each time you inhale.

5. Keep your attitude passive; disregard thoughts that drift in.

6. Continue for 10 to 20 minutes once or twice a day.

You can pick almost any focus word or phrase, such as the word "one." Some meditators find it helpful to focus on the breath—in, out, in, out—rather than on a word or phrase. Others prefer to focus on an object, such as a candle flame. If you want to time your session, peek at a watch or clock occasionally, but don't set a jarring alarm. Getting to your feet immediately after a session can make you feel slightly dizzy, so sit quietly for a few moments first with your eyes closed. The technique works best on an empty stomach, either before a meal or about 2 hours after eating. Avoid those times when you are obviously tired unless you want to fall asleep. Although you will feel refreshed after the first session, it may take a month or more to get noticeable results, such as lower blood pressure.

After trying the two relaxation techniques in Activities 1 and 2 (progressive muscle relaxation; relaxation response) several times each, which do you prefer?

_____

Why?

_____

_____

Use your preferred relaxation technique daily over a 2-week period of time. Identify for each day your location, approximate length of time taken, and your feelings when finished.

Your preferred method: _____

	Date:	Date:	Date:	Date:	Date:	Date:	Date:
Location							
Length							
Feelings: calm, relaxed, etc.							

	Date:	Date:	Date:	Date:	Date:	Date:	Date:
Location							
Length							
Feelings: calm, relaxed, etc.							

Name: _____ Course Number: _____

Section: _____ Date: _____

Creative Problem Solving

Activity 1: Scenarios

Directions

Choose one of the following problems. This activity can provide good practice for the times when you will need to apply these skills to real life.

Problem 1: Paul is called into his supervisor's office and told that the company must lay off some employees. Paul will be laid off in 2 months. He is married and has two small children. He has a mortgage payment on his home and a car payment each month.

Problem 2: You are upset after having an argument with your junior high school–aged son about the trouble he is getting into at school.

Problem 3: Maria has four final exams and only 2 days left to study for them. She is anxious because she doesn't think she will have enough time to study for the exams.

Which of the problems did you choose? _____

1. Define the problem.

   _____

   _____

   _____

2. List the facts.

   _____

   _____

3. List possible solutions (at least four).

   a. _____

   _____

   b. _____

   _____

   c. _____

   _____

   d. _____

   _____

4. Analyze and evaluate the possible solutions.

_____

_____

_____

5. Select one solution to implement.

_____

_____

_____

6. Evaluate the results (for this assignment, give ways you would evaluate).

_____

_____

_____

Activity 2: Problem-Solving Steps

Write a problem that was or is stressing you. Go through the problem-solving steps. Write the problem:

_____

_____

_____

1. Define the problem.

_____

_____

_____

2. List the facts.

_____

_____

_____

3. List possible solutions (at least four).

a. _____

_____

_____

b. _____

_____

_____

c. _____

_____

_____

d. _____

_____

_____

4. Analyze and evaluate the possible solutions.

_____

_____

_____

5. Select one solution to implement.

_____

_____

_____

6. Evaluate the results (for this assignment give ways you would evaluate).

_____

_____

_____

Name: _____ Course Number: _____

Section: _____ Date: _____

Chapter 10: Critical Thinking Questions

Mental Health and Coping with Stress

1. Jackson was able to determine that exercising helped relieve the speech anxiety he was having. Review Figure 10.5 and Figure 10.6 in the textbook. Are you experiencing any of the harmful stress symptoms listed? If so, do you think stress is the cause? If yes, what are the specific stressors? What physical activities might you do to help relieve these stressors?

2. Review your list of life stress sources. Next to each source, list whether you would use environmental engineering, mind engineering, or physical engineering to manage the stressor. Would more than one strategy be useful? Do you see physical activity helping to manage the stress in your life? Why or why not?

3. Stressors can be a result of situations present on your campus or in your campus community. Community stressors may be problems such as crime, pollution, lack of recreation facilities, and overcrowded classrooms or residence halls. Identify what you consider to be a major stressor in your campus community. How would you go about changing this stressor?

_____

_____

_____

_____

_____

_____

_____

_____

_____

_____

_____

_____

Critical Thinking Questions

Name: _____ Course Number: _____

Section: _____ Date: _____

Alcohol Use Disorders Identification Test (AUDIT)

Is the way or amount I drink harming my health? Should I cut down on my drinking? Taking the following assessment will help you answer these questions.

Please circle the answer that is correct for you.

1. How often do you have a drink containing alcohol?

Never	Monthly or less	Two to four times a month	Two to three times per week	Four or more times a week

2. How many drinks containing alcohol do you have on a typical day when you are drinking?

1 or 2	3 or 4	5 or 6	7 or 9	10 or more

3. How often do you have six or more drinks on one occasion?

Never	Less than monthly	Monthly	Two to three times per week	Four or more times a week

4. How often during the last year have you found that you were not able to stop drinking once you had started?

Never	Less than monthly	Monthly	Two to three times per week	Four or more times a week

5. How often during the last year have you failed to do what was normally expected from you because of drinking?

Never	Less than monthly	Monthly	Two to three times per week	Four or more times a week

6. How often during the last year have you needed a first drink in the morning to get yourself going after a heavy drinking session?

Never	Less than monthly	Monthly	Two to three times per week	Four or more times a week

7. How often during the last year have you had a feeling of guilt or remorse after drinking?

Never	Less than monthly	Monthly	Two to three times per week	Four or more times a week

8. How often during the last year have you been unable to remember what happened the night before because you had been drinking?

| Never | Less than monthly | Monthly | Two to three times per week | Four or more times a week |

9. Have you or someone else been injured as a result of your drinking?

| No | Yes, but not in the last year | Yes, during the last year |

10. Has a relative or friend, or a doctor or other health worker, been concerned about your drinking or suggested you cut down?

| No | Yes, but not in the last year | Yes, during the last year |

Correlate your answers to the scores in the table below, and then compute your score by adding up the numbers.

Answer Key					
Question	**Answer #1**	**Answer #2**	**Answer #3**	**Answer #4**	**Answer #5**
1	0	1	2	3	4
2	0	1	2	3	4
3	0	1	2	3	4
4	0	1	2	3	4
5	0	1	2	3	4
6	0	1	2	3	4
7	0	1	2	3	4
8	0	1	2	3	4
9	0	2	4		
10	0	2	4		

Your score: _____

What Your Score Means

If you scored 8 or more points, your drinking habits may not be safe or healthy for yourself or others. Limit how much you drink or quit altogether.

BELOW 8: You probably don't have a diagnosable alcohol problem, but, if you are concerned about how alcohol is affecting you, you should make changes.

8 to 11: You may very well have reasons to be concerned.

11 to 15: There are some serious indications that your drinking is a problem.

ABOVE 15: You most likely have a drinking problem.

Source: Reproduced from Alcohol Alert (2005). Screening for Alcohol Use and Alcohol-Related Problems. National Institutes on Health, National Institute on Alcohol Abuse and Alcoholism. Online: http://pubs.niaaa.nih.gov/publications/aa65/aa65.htm.

Name: _____ Course Number: _____

Section: _____ Date: _____

Why Do You Smoke?

Here are some statements made by people to describe what they get out of smoking cigarettes. How often do you feel this way when smoking? Circle one number for each statement.

Important: Answer every question.

	Always	Frequently	Occasionally	Seldom	Never
A. I smoke cigarettes to keep myself from slowing down.	5	4	3	2	1
B. Handling a cigarette is part of the enjoyment of smoking it.	5	4	3	2	1
C. Smoking cigarettes is pleasant and relaxing.	5	4	3	2	1
D. I light up a cigarette when I feel angry about something.	5	4	3	2	1
E. When I have run out of cigarettes I find it almost unbearable until I can get them.	5	4	3	2	1
F. I smoke cigarettes automatically without even being aware of it.	5	4	3	2	1
G. I smoke cigarettes to stimulate me, to perk myself up.	5	4	3	2	1
H. Part of the enjoyment of smoking a cigarette comes from the steps I take to light up.	5	4	3	2	1
I. I find cigarettes pleasurable.	5	4	3	2	1
J. When I feel uncomfortable or upset about something, I light up a cigarette.	5	4	3	2	1
K. I am very much aware of the fact when I am not smoking a cigarette.	5	4	3	2	1
L. I light up a cigarette without realizing I still have one burning in the ashtray.	5	4	3	2	1
M. I smoke cigarettes to give me a lift.	5	4	3	2	1
N. When I smoke a cigarette, part of the enjoyment is watching the smoke as I exhale it.	5	4	3	2	1

	Always	Frequently	Occasionally	Seldom	Never
O. I want a cigarette most when I am comfortable and relaxed.	5	4	3	2	1
P. When I feel blue, or want to take my mind off cares and worries, I smoke cigarettes.	5	4	3	2	1
Q. I get a real gnawing hunger for a cigarette when I haven't smoked for a while.	5	4	3	2	1
R. I've found a cigarette in my mouth and I didn't remember putting it there.	5	4	3	2	1

How to Score

1. Enter the numbers you have circled in the following spaces, putting the number you have circled to Question A over line A, to Question B over line B, and so forth.

2. Add the three scores on each line to get your totals. For example, the sum of your scores over lines A, G, and M gives you your score on Stimulation, lines B, H, and N give the score on Handling, and so on.

Totals

____		____		____			____
A	+	G	+	M	=		Stimulation
B	+	H	+	N	=		Handling
C	+	I	+	O	=		Pleasurable relaxation
D	+	J	+	P	=		Crutch; tension reduction
E	+	K	+	Q	=		Craving: psychological addiction
F	+	L	+	R	=		Habit

Scores of 11 or above indicate that this factor is an important source of satisfaction for the smoker. Scores of 7 or less are low and probably indicate that this factor does not apply to you. Scores in between are marginal.

Source: Reproduced from Smoker's Self-Testing Kit developed by Daniel Horn, PhD. Originally published by National Clearinghouse for Smoking and Health, Department of Health, Education, and Welfare.

Name: _____ Course Number: _____

Section: _____ Date: _____

The Drugs You Take

Step 1: Keep a Drug Diary

List the drugs you consume daily over the course of a week. Did you drink coffee? List the number of cups. How about energy drinks or caffeinated sodas? Tea? Did you smoke cigarettes? How many? Did you drink alcohol? Did you take over-the-counter medications? Prescription medications? Also make note of your stress level and mood at the time you used each drug.

Example:

Day	Substance	Amount	Drug	What did it do for you?	Stress level 1 = low stress 2 = moderate stress 3 = high stress	Mood (e.g., angry, happy, hopeful, depressed, bored, frustrated)
1	Red Bull Energy drink	1 can	Caffeine	Helped me wake up	3	Frustrated
	Advil	2 tablets	Ibuprofen	Relief from body ache	2	Indifferent

Your Drug Diary:

Day	Substance	Amount	Drug	What did it do for you?	Stress level 1 = low stress 2 = moderate stress 3 = high stress	Mood (e.g., angry, happy, depressed, bored)
1						
2						
3						
4						
5						
6						
7						

Step 2: Review and Reflect on Your Drug Diary

Answer the following questions as they relate to your 1-week drug diary.

1. Were you surprised about anything from your drug diary? _____ If yes, what surprised you?

   _____

2. Did you notice any patterns in your use of drugs? _____ If yes, what patterns were apparent?

   _____

3. Are you using any drugs as a coping mechanism to deal with your stress levels or moods? _____ If yes, which drugs?

   _____

4. Looking at your drug diary, are there any substances you would like to reduce or eliminate? _____

Name: _____ Course Number: _____

Section: _____ Date: _____

Concerned About Someone?

"I am concerned about someone who uses alcohol and/or drugs." According to the National Council on Alcoholism and Drug Dependence, Inc. (NCADD), you should ask the following questions.

Question	Yes	No
1. Do you worry about how much your friend or loved one uses alcohol or drugs?		
2. Do you lie or make excuses about their behavior when they drink or use drugs?		
3. Do they get angry with you if you try to discuss their drinking or drug use?		
4. Have you ever been hurt or embarrassed by their behavior when they're drunk, stoned, or strung-out?		
5. Do you have concerns about how much time and money they spend on alcohol and drugs?		
6. Do you resent having to pick up their responsibilities because they are drunk, high, or hungover?		
7. Do you ever get scared or nervous about their behavior when they're drinking or using drugs?		
8. Do you ever feel like you're losing it—"going crazy"—just really stressed out?		
9. Have you ever considered calling the police because of their alcohol or drug use or their behavior while under the influence?		

Source: Reproduced from National Council on Alcoholism and Drug Dependence, Inc. (2012). Concerned about someone? Online: http://www.ncadd.org/index.php/for-youth/concerned-about-someone.

If you answered "yes" to any of these nine questions, you may want to talk to your friend or loved one right away. You may also want to see a health professional specifically trained and experienced in dealing with alcohol and drugs for help. A great place to start is on your campus. Most college campuses have a student health center or counseling center staffed with health professionals who can support your friend in cutting back or quitting drug use. In addition, you can find a drug abuse treatment program with the Substance Abuse Treatment Facility Locator at http://findtreatment.samhasa.gov. This searchable directory of drug and alcohol treatment programs shows the location of facilities around the country that treat drug misuse and abuse problems. You can also visit the National Council on Alcoholism and Drug Dependence (NCADD) website at www.ncadd.org or call 1-800-622-2255 for assistance.

About the NCADD: The National Council on Alcoholism and Drug Dependence, Inc., and its Affiliate Network is a voluntary health organization dedicated to fighting the nation's #1 health problem—alcoholism, drug addiction, and the devastating consequences of alcohol and other drugs on individuals, families, and communities.

Name: _____   Course Number: _____

Section: _____   Date: _____

Chapter 11: Critical Thinking Questions

Making Informed Decisions About Drug Use

1. "I really don't like the taste of liquor that much, but after the first couple of shots, it doesn't taste all that bad. I know I shouldn't drink and I always have a hangover the next day, but, hey, college is stressful and how else can I deal with the stress of getting the grades to keep my scholarship and making my parents happy?" What's your opinion of this person's attitude? Explain why you agree or disagree. If you disagree, how do you think this person can deal with the stress of getting good grades?

2. College campuses often accept money from companies that sell alcoholic beverages—to support athletic events, for example. By allowing these companies to advertise at campus events, the university makes considerable money to enhance the campus environment and provide quality education. What is your campus's policy on allowing alcohol companies to advertise or sponsor events on campus? Do you agree or disagree with this policy?

3. Purchase a popular magazine and count the number of cigarette ads in the issue. In reviewing each of the ads, respond to the following questions:

   a. Who is the ad targeting (young people, older adults, women)?

   b. How is the ad appealing to the target audience (fun, sex)?

   c. What does the ad seem to promise if you smoke their brand of cigarette?

   _____

   _____

   _____

   _____

   _____

   _____

   _____

   _____

   _____

   _____

Critical Thinking Questions

Name: _____   Course Number: _____

Section: _____   Date: _____

Skeptical Buyer Exercise

Locate an advertisement selling an exercise product (such as an infomercial or magazine advertisement) and answer the following questions.

1. What is the name of the product?

_____

2. What is the purported purpose of the product?

_____

3. What marketing strategies are being used to persuade you to purchase the product? See Table 12.1 in *Physical Activity & Health, Fourth Edition.*

_____

_____

_____

4. In your opinion, is the product worth what the company is selling it for?

_____

_____

_____

5. What portions of the marketing strategy are suspect?

_____

_____

_____

6. Would you buy the product? Why or why not?

_____

_____

_____

Name: _____ Course Number: _____

Section: _____ Date: _____

ACSM Health and Fitness Facility Evaluation

The American College of Sports Medicine has guidelines for selecting and effectively using a health and fitness facility. Visit a local health and fitness facility and answer the following questions.

Health and Fitness Facility _____

Before joining, take a tour and ask the following questions:	Yes	No
Does the facility offer the type of exercise or program in which you are interested?		
Do qualified exercise instructors develop the programs?		
Will staff members modify the programs to meet your needs?		
Does the facility offer programs to address medical conditions?		
Does the facility offer programs for the age group in which you are interested?		
Does the facility offer fitness assessments and a personalized exercise program or prescription?		
Check for these safety features:	**Yes**	**No**
Does the facility have a posted emergency response evacuation plan?		
Is staff qualified to execute the emergency response evacuation plan?		
Does the facility have automated external defibrillators (AEDs) on site?		
Is the facility clean and well maintained?		
Is the facility free from physical or environmental hazards?		
Is the facility appropriately lit?		
Does the facility have adequate heating, cooling, and ventilation?		
Does the facility have adequate parking?		
Check to see if the facility provides for or adheres to the following:	**Yes**	**No**
Does the facility offer a preactivity screening, such as the PAR-Q, to assess whether members have medical conditions or risk factors that should be addressed by a physician?		
Aside from an initial general health and wellness screening, does the facility have a health and fitness screening method appropriate for the type of exercise you will undertake?		
Does the facility offer fitness assessments?		

Check to make sure the entire staff has credentials and education from credible institutions:	Yes	No
Do staff members have appropriate education, certification, and training that is recognized by the industry and the public as representing a high level of competence and credibility?		
Is there sufficient staff on site?		
Are staff members easy to recognize?		
Are the staff members friendly and helpful?		
Do staff members receive ongoing professional training?		
Do staff members provide each new member with an orientation to the equipment and/or facility?		
Are the staff members trained in CPR, in the use of AEDs, and in first aid?		
Are the staff members knowledgeable about your health conditions?		
Can the staff help you set realistic exercise goals?		
Before signing a contract, consider the following:	**Yes**	**No**
Does the staff pressure you into purchasing a membership?		
Does the membership fee fit into your budget?		
Is there a trial membership program?		
Is there a grace period during which you can cancel your membership and receive a refund?		
Are there different membership options and are all the fees for services posted?		
Does the facility provide you with a written set of rules and policies, which govern the responsibilities of members as well as the facility?		
Does the facility have a procedure to inform members of any changes in charges, services, or policies?		

Source: Reprinted with permission of the American College of Sports Medicine. Copyright © 2011 American College of Sports Medicine. These questions were taken from a brochure created and updated by Hank Williford, EdD, FACSM, and Michelle Olson, PhD, FACSM, and they are a product of ACSM's Consumer Information Committee. Visit ACSM online at www.acsm.org.

Would you join this health and fitness facility? Why or why not?

_____

_____

Name: _____ Course Number: _____

Section: _____ Date: _____

Test Your Supplement Savvy

Advertised through the media, displayed in grocery stores and pharmacies, and promoted widely on the Internet, dietary supplements can look just like other consumer products on the shelf. But are they? Take this quiz to find out how much you know about using dietary supplements safely.

1. A supplement labeled "natural" means that it also is:

   1. Mild

   2. Without any risk of side effects

   3. Safe to use with other medications

   4. None of the above

2. Because dietary supplements are so readily available—and don't require a doctor's prescription—they are much safer than drug products and can be used to self-treat illnesses without a health professional's advice or supervision.

   True or False

3. Testimonials in dietary supplement promotions give a good idea of the supplement's benefits and safety because they're based on firsthand accounts.

   True or False

4. Many supplements have proven health benefits.

   True or False

5. Before you start taking a dietary supplement, you should talk it over with a knowledgeable person like:

   1. Your doctor or health professional

   2. Your pharmacist

   3. A supplement salesperson

   4. A friend who takes the supplement

Answers to Test Your Supplement Savvy

1. **D.** The term "natural" may suggest to consumers that the supplement is safe, especially when compared with prescription drugs that are known to have side effects, but natural is not necessarily safe. Although many supplements can be used safely by most people, other supplements, including some herbal products, can be dangerous. Aristolochic acid, which has been found in some traditional Chinese herbal remedies, has been linked to severe kidney disease. And the herb comfrey contains certain alkaloids that, when ingested, have been linked to serious, even fatal, liver damage. Animal studies suggest that the herb may cause cancer too. Even certain vitamins can be toxic at high doses. And certain supplements have been found to interact with other medications in ways that could cause injury.

2. **False.** Studies have shown that some herbal products interact with drugs and can have a wide range of effects. For example, St. John's Wort can lower the effects of indinavir, a protease inhibitor for treating HIV. St. John's Wort also may interfere with drugs used by organ transplant patients and drugs used to treat depression, seizures, and certain cancers. In addition, there are concerns that it may reduce the effectiveness of oral contraceptives. Garlic, ginkgo, danshen, and dong quai can cause blood to thin, which could cause serious problems for people on drugs like warfarin or aspirin. Dietary supplements are not required to go through the same premarket government review for quality, safety, and efficacy as drug products. But that doesn't mean they should be taken lightly—or without consulting your health care professional, especially if you have a medical condition or are taking other drugs.

3. **False.** It's unwise to judge a product's efficacy or safety based only on testimonials. First, it is very difficult to verify the accuracy of the account: some marketers may embellish or even make up testimonials to sell their product. Second, you can't generalize one person's experience to others. Anecdotes are not a substitute for valid science.

4. **True.** Studies suggest that several popular supplements, including herbal products, may provide health benefits. For example, calcium can reduce the risk of osteoporosis, folic acid during pregnancy can prevent birth defects, and there is some evidence suggesting that St. John's Wort may be helpful for some people with mild depression. Verify any health claims with a reliable source, such as the National Institutes of Health's Office of Dietary Supplements, a public health or scientific organization like the American Cancer Society or the Arthritis Foundation, and your health provider.

5. **A or B.** Talk to your doctor, pharmacist, or other health provider about any medicines you take, as well as any dietary supplements you're using or thinking about using. Though some doctors have limited knowledge of herbal products and other supplements, they have access to the most current research and can help monitor your condition to ensure that no problems develop or serious interactions occur. Retailers or marketers can be good sources of information about their products and their ingredients, but bear in mind that they have a financial interest in their products. If your doctor or pharmacist has a financial interest in the product, get a second, independent opinion.

Source: Reproduced from the Federal Trade Commission (2001). You're supplement savvy. Online: http://www.ftc.gov/bcp/edu/pubs/consumer/health/hea09.shtm.

Name: ——————————————————————— Course Number: ———————————————

Section: ——————————————————————— Date: ———————————————

Chapter 12: Critical Thinking Questions

Health Consumerism

1. Like Toni, you are constantly bombarded with advertisements about a diet pill or drink that will guarantee losing *X* pounds per week. These advertisements are often displayed on college and university campuses. As you walk to class, take a look around to see if you notice any of these advertisements. Record what you see. Also, review the most recent issue of your college or university newspaper. Are there any ads for fad diets or pills? If so, who are they targeting?

2. In a popular magazine, find an advertisement that you believe might be misleading or fraudulent. Determine which of the advertising approaches are used to convince readers to purchase the product. What argument would you present to counter the advertising claims?

3. Speculate about why people often fall victim to common physical activity and health misconceptions, frauds, or fallacies.

4. As a critical health consumer, where would you suggest peers go to find valid information on physical activity and health? Give three sources and explain how you determined they were valid.

——

——

——

——

——

——

——

——

——

——

——

© 2014 Jones & Bartlett Learning

Critical Thinking Questions

Name: ———————————————————— Course Number: ————————————

Section: ———————————————————— Date: ————————————

Thinking About Your "Relationship Portfolio"

There are several things to consider in a relationship portfolio, including the type of each relationship, the number of people in it, the time spent in those relationships, and the quality of each relationship. Much like a financial investment portfolio for retirement, diversifying (or expanding) and reflecting on your relationship portfolio is important.

Complete the following relationship portfolio chart based on the following types of relationships: acquaintances/casual friends, work/school relationships, internet-based relationships, family, best friends, and romantic partners.

Types of Relationships	Acquaintances/ Casual Friends	Work/ School	Internet-Based	Family	Best Friends	Romantic Partners
Number of relationships						
Time (per day) spent in relationships						
Quality of relationships+						

+Importance scale: 1 = unimportant; 2 = somewhat important; 3 = important; 4 = very important

Reflection Activity

Each type of relationship can play a valuable and different role in our lives. Take some time to reflect on your relationship portfolio by answering the following questions.

1. Are you weighted too heavily in one relationship category?

———————————————————————————————

———————————————————————————————

———————————————————————————————

2. Are you missing some important relationships that you wish you had?

———————————————————————————————

———————————————————————————————

———————————————————————————————

3. Compare the amount of time you spend in each type of relationship with the importance of the relationship type to you. Do you want to make any adjustments? For example, do you want to spend more time in some of your relationships, or do you want more relationships in a particular category?

_____

_____

_____

4. What adjustments might you consider making to the quantity, quality, or amount of time spent in your relationships?

_____

_____

_____

Small Group Activity

Consider how many close or best friends you would like. How much time do you want to spend with your best friends? Discuss the following questions about close friendships in your small groups.

1. How can I develop close friendships and ways to meet new people? Share why you think close relationships are important.

_____

_____

2. What circumstances prompt you to call on your close relationships (e.g., best friends, family, romantic partners)?

_____

_____

3. For what types of things do you seek support? For example, who do you call when you do not do well on a test? Who do you call for support if you have an argument with another friend or a family member?

_____

_____

4. What types of things do you feel comfortable sharing with your acquaintances/casual friends?

_____

_____

Name: _____ Course Number: _____

Section: _____ Date: _____

How Much Do You Know About Healthy Relationships?

The answers are given on the next page.

1. A healthy way to show that you are listening to someone is to:

    a. Say: "It seems like you're saying you would like me to call you if I'm going to be late."

    b. Look the person in the eye when he or she is speaking.

    c. Wait until the other person has finished speaking before you say something.

    d. All of the above

2. If you want to talk with your friend about something private, which is the best way to do this?

    a. Demand to speak with your friend right away when he or she is in a big group of people.

    b. Find your friend when he or she is alone so that you can talk privately together.

    c. Don't say anything because it's better to hold your feelings inside.

    d. Stop talking to your friend until he or she asks what's wrong.

3. A healthy way to show your hurt feelings is by saying which of the following statements?

    a. "You make me mad when you do that."

    b. "I hate you when you don't do what I want."

    c. "I feel upset when you do that."

    d. "You should know what I'm feeling."

4. If you and a good friend are having an argument that you can't seem to work out, what should you do?

    a. Tell your friend that you won't talk to her or him until she or he says you're right.

    b. Talk behind her or his back with all your other friends.

    c. Ask a trusted adult for help.

    d. Storm out of the room and slam the door behind you.

5. If you and a good friend are going through a tough time, it might help you to do which of the following?

    a. Ignore your friend and spend all your time with other people.

    b. Blame all the problems on yourself.

    c. Stop listening to what the other person has to say.

    d. Remember that you care about each other and try to listen extra hard to each other.

6. What is one way to know if friends really care about you?

    a. They like that you help them with their math homework all the time.

    b. They are happy for you when you do well.

    c. They don't say they are sorry if they hurt your feelings because friends don't have to apologize.

    d. They like to give you advice so that you do things the way they do them.

7. Which one of these will not help you make new friends?

    a. Introducing yourself and remembering people's names

    b. Not joining a new club because you are not sure you will like it

    c. Getting involved in after-school activities

    d. Being sensitive to other people's feelings

8. What should you do if your friends pressure you to drink?

    a. Be strong and say, "I don't want to."

    b. Spend time with other friends who don't pressure you, and also make new friends.

    c. Suggest other things that you and your friends can do for fun.

    d. All of the above

Answers to How Much Do You Know About Healthy Relationships?

1. D. Having good listening skills is very important for all relationships. One way to show someone that you are listening is to repeat what was said so you do not misunderstand him or her. Looking at a person when he or she is talking to you and not interrupting are two additional ways to show you are listening.

2. B. The best idea is to speak with your friend alone. You may want to quietly pull your friend aside and arrange a later time to speak in private. In a healthy relationship, it is important to share your feelings. If you are having trouble talking to your friend about something, think about talking to a trusted adult.

3. C. A good way to show your feelings is by using "I statements." Voicing your feelings this way helps you to be direct, honest, and positive instead of blaming others. In order to have healthy relationships, you need to tell people how you are feeling. No one can read your mind, even if they are really close to you! Try using statements such as, "I feel mad/sad/upset/etc. when you don't listen to me."

4. **C.** Sometimes you may find that an argument is getting nowhere and you and your friend may need help from a trusted adult. Talk with someone who won't take sides so she or he can listen to what you both have to say. You may find that sitting down together with an adult will help you to organize your thoughts so you can work things out.

5. **D.** Even in healthy relationships, people disagree and argue. Difficult times may pass if you are able to talk about your feelings with one another. Healthy relationships take time and energy.

6. **B.** Your true friends want you to be happy and are happy for you when things go your way. If someone only likes you because you help them, doesn't say he or she is sorry for hurting your feelings, or always wants you to do things their way, this person is not a true friend.

7. **B.** Here are some great ways to help you make new friends: Introduce yourself and try to remember people's names, get involved in after-school activities, and be sensitive to other people's feelings. New friends will appreciate all of these things!

8. **D.** All of these options are good choices to help you handle a pressure-filled situation involving alcohol.

Source: Reproduced from U.S. Department of Health and Human Services. Office on Women's Health. Online: http://www.girlshealth.gov/relationships/quizzes/quiz.relknow.cfm.

Name: _____   Course Number: _____

Section: _____   Date: _____

How Much Do You Know About Ways to Deal with Conflict?

The answers are given on the next page.

1. If you're feeling angry, what should you do?

   a. Stomp around the room but say nothing.

   b. Slam the door, hard.

   c. Ignore your friend at school.

   d. Carefully tell your friend what you are feeling.

2. By not dealing with conflict in a healthy way, what could happen?

   a. You could lose a good friend.

   b. You could be treated unfairly at work or school.

   c. You could not get something you want or need.

   d. You might feel like you can never make things better.

   e. All of the above

3. True or False: Counting to 10 before speaking if you're feeling angry is a healthy way of dealing with conflict.

   a. True

   b. False

4. Which statement can help people stay open and honest when there is a conflict?

   a. "You only think about yourself!"

   b. "I feel upset when you don't ask me what I want to do."

   c. "You don't care about me!"

   d. "You will never be happy with my homework!"

5. How can you stay safe from violence?

   a. Choose your friends carefully.

   b. Report any weapons to a trusted adult.

   c. Practice "safety in numbers."

   d. All of the above

   e. None of the above

6. True or False: Staying calm during a disagreement with your parents can help show them that you are growing up.

    a. True

    b. False

7. True or False: You should never compromise when you are mad at someone.

    a. True

    b. False

Answers to How Much Do You Know About Ways to Deal with Conflict?

1. D. If you're feeling angry, you should carefully tell your friend what you are feeling.

2. E. By not dealing with conflict in a healthy way, you could lose a good friend, be treated unfairly at work or school, not get something you want or need, and/or feel like you can never make things better.

3. A. Counting to 10 before speaking if you're feeling angry is a healthy way of dealing with conflict.

4. B. A great way of letting someone know how you feel is to use an "I statement" and to state your true feelings, such as "I feel upset when you don't ask me what I want to do."

5. D. To stay safe from violence choose your friends carefully, report any weapons to a trusted adult, and practice "safety in numbers."

6. A. Staying calm during a disagreement with your parents can help show them that you are growing up.

7. B. You should compromise when you are mad at someone.

Source: Reproduced from U.S. Department of Health and Human Services. Office on Women's Health. Online: http://www.girlshealth.gov/relationships/quizzes/quiz.conflict.cfm.

After completing Activity 13.3, ask yourself if there is room for growth in your relationships or in the way you deal with conflict. Answer these questions, and then discuss them in small groups.

1. For you, what makes it hard to address conflict directly for you?

2. Are there times when certain people with whom you find it harder or easier to address conflict?

3. What goals do you have for improving the way you deal with conflict?

Name: _____ Course Number: _____

Section: _____ Date: _____

Am I in an Abusive Relationship?

Does Your Partner . . .

Embarrass you with put-downs?	Yes	No
Look at you or act in ways that scare you?	Yes	No
Control what you do, who you see or talk to, or where you go?	Yes	No
Stop you from seeing your friends or family members?	Yes	No
Take your money or Social Security check, make you ask for money, or refuse to give you money?	Yes	No
Make all of the decisions?	Yes	No
Tell you that you're a bad parent or threaten to take away or hurt your children?	Yes	No
Prevent you from working or attending school?	Yes	No
Act like the abuse is no big deal, it's your fault, or even deny doing it?	Yes	No
Destroy your property or threaten to kill your pets?	Yes	No
Intimidate you with guns, knives, or other weapons?	Yes	No
Shove you, slap you, choke you, or hit you?	Yes	No
Force you to try to drop charges?	Yes	No
Threaten to commit suicide?	Yes	No
Threaten to kill you?	Yes	No

If you answered yes to even one of these questions, you may be in an abusive relationship.

For support and more information, please call the National Domestic Violence Hotline at 1-800-799-SAFE (7233) or TTY 1-800-787-3224.

Be Safe. Computer use can be monitored and is impossible to completely clear. If you are afraid your Internet and/or computer usage might be monitored, please use a safer computer, call your local hotline, and/or call the National Domestic Violence Hotline at 1-800-799-SAFE (7233) or TTY 1-800-787-3224.

Source: Reproduced from National Domestic Violence Hotline. Online: www.thehotline.org/is-this-abuse/am-I-being-abused-Z. Contact The Hotline by phone at 1-800-799-SAFE (7233) or 1-800-787-3224 (TTY).

Name: _____ Course Number: _____

Section: _____ Date: _____

Chapter 13: Critical Thinking Questions

Developing Healthy Social and Intimate Relationships

1. Read the following scenario and identify several communication problems. How could Bob and Sandy have handled this situation using healthy communication skills?

   Bob: Well, Sandy, you know that this weekend is the big reunion of all my fraternity brothers, and I'd like you to join me in celebrating our 100-year anniversary!

   Sandy: Now you ask! I've already told my theater group that we would join them for their weekend outing.

   Bob: Great, you didn't even ask me, you just went ahead and made plans for me this weekend!

   Sandy: Ask you? You have been so busy lately with work and school, I haven't even had a chance to talk to you let alone ask you if you wanted to spend the weekend with me and the theater group.

   Bob: Oh great, now it is my fault that I've been working so hard and trying to get good grades. Go ahead, blame it on me!

   Sandy: Okay! It's your fault we never spend any time together. I'm sick of this! What will it be, your fraternity brothers or me?

   Bob: Well, now I'm having to choose between you and my fraternity brothers. That's easy! My fraternity brothers any day—at least they understand how hard it is to work and go to school!

2. "An intimate relationship may be sexual, but a sexual relationship is not necessarily an intimate one." Discuss the difference(s) between an intimate relationship and a sexual relationship.

3. Identify 10 terms that are gender-biased. Example: fireman.

4. Identify five television shows that have characters in stereotypical male or female roles. Identify the characters and briefly explain the roles they play.

5. Do you and/or your romantic partner wish to increase your level of communication? If so, what steps might you take to do so?

6. Identify at least three ways that healthy relationships can improve your physical health. How are your relationships contributing to your physical health?

7. Discuss the positives and negatives of having online friendships.

8. What are some of the risks of text messaging something important?

9. Identify some movies or television shows in which there was a conflict between two close friends or romantic partners. Discuss what they may have been able to do differently to deal with the conflict and improve their communication.

_____

_____

_____

_____

_____

_____

_____

_____

_____

_____

_____

_____

_____

_____

_____

_____

_____

_____

_____

_____

_____

_____

_____

_____

_____

Name: _____ Course Number: _____

Section: _____ Date: _____

Are You at an Increased Risk for Having a Heart Attack?

There are a number of factors that can lead to heart disease. To decide which factors to focus on, first you should compute YOUR personal cardiac risk. Here is a quick self-assessment quiz to determine your risk for a heart attack.

Factor	Yes	No	Don't Know
Do you smoke?			
Is your blood pressure 140/90 mmHg or higher, *or* have you been told by a doctor that your blood pressure is high?			
Has your doctor told you that your LDL ("bad") cholesterol is too high, *or* that your total cholesterol level is 200 mg/dL *or* higher, *or* that your HDL ("good") cholesterol is less than 40 mg/dL?			
Has your father or brother had a heart attack before age 55, *or* has your mother or sister had one before age 65?			
Do you have diabetes OR a fasting blood sugar of 126 mg/dL or higher, *or* do you need medication to control your blood sugar?			
Are you a man over 45 years of age?			
Are you a woman over 55 years of age?			
Do you have a body mass index (BMI) score of 25 or more?			
Do you get less than a total of 30 minutes of physical activity on most days?			
Has a doctor told you that you have angina (chest pains), or have had a heart attack?			

If you answered "yes" to any of the statements, you are at an increased risk for having a heart attack. If you don't know some of the answers, check with your health care provider.

Source: Reproduced from National Heart, Lung, and Blood Institute (NHLBI), National Institutes of Health (NIH). (2007). Are You at an Increased Risk of Having a Heart Attack? Online: http://www.nhlbi.nih.gov/actintime/haws/quiz.htm.

Name: _____ Course Number: _____

Section: _____ Date: _____

Risk Assessment Tool for Estimating Your 10-Year Risk for Having a Heart Attack

In general, the higher your LDL level and the more risk factors you have (other than LDL), the greater your chances are of developing heart disease or having a heart attack. Some people are at high risk for a heart attack because they already have heart disease. Other people are at high risk for developing heart problems because they have diabetes (which is a strong risk factor) or a combination of risk factors for heart disease. The risk assessment tool for having a heart attack uses information from the Framingham Heart Study to predict a person's chance of having a heart attack in the next 10 years. This tool is designed for adults aged 20 and older with heart disease or diabetes. Follow these steps to determine your risk for developing heart disease.

Step 1: In the following table, check each of the listed risk factors you have; these are risk factors that affect your LDL goal.

Major Risk Factors	Yes
Cigarette smoking	
High blood pressure (140/90 mmHg or higher or on blood pressure medication)	
Low HDL cholesterol (less than 40 mg/dL)*	
Family history of early heart disease (heart disease in father or brother before age 55; heart disease in mother or sister before age 65)	
Age (men 45 years or older; women 55 years or older)	

*If your HDL cholesterol is 60 mg/dL or higher, subtract 1 from your total count.

Even though obesity and physical activity are not counted in this list, they are conditions that need to be corrected.

Step 2: How many major risk factors do you have? _____ If you have 2 or more risk factors from Step 1, use the Framingham Point Scores in the following table to find your risk score. Risk score refers to the chance of having a heart attack in the next 10 years and is given as a percentage.

My risk score is _____percent.

Estimate of 10-Year Risk for Men*

*Data in the tables that follow reproduced from National Heart, Lung, and Blood Institute (NHLBI); National Institutes of Health (NIH). (2005). NIH Publication No. 05–3290.

Framingham Point Scores by Age Group

Age	Points
20–34	−9
35–39	−4
40–44	0
45–49	3
50–54	6
55–59	8
60–64	10
65–69	11
70–74	12
75–79	13

Framingham Point Scores by Age Group and Total Cholesterol

Total Cholesterol	Age 20–39	Age 40–49	Age 50–59	Age 60–69	Age 70–79
< 160	0	0	0	0	0
160–199	4	3	2	1	0
200–239	7	5	3	1	0
240–279	9	6	4	2	1
280+	11	8	5	3	1

Framingham Point Scores by Age Group and Smoking Status

	Age 20–39	Age 40–49	Age 50–59	Age 60–69	Age 70–79
Nonsmoker	0	0	0	0	0
Smoker	8	5	3	1	1

Framingham Point Scores by HDL Level

HDL	Points
60+	−1
50–59	0
40–49	1
< 40	2

Risk Assessment Tool for Estimating Your 10-Year Risk for Having a Heart Attack

Framingham Point Scores by Systolic Blood Pressure and Treatment Status

Systolic BP	If Untreated	If Treated
< 120	0	0
120–129	0	1
130–139	1	2
140–159	1	2
160+	2	3

10-Year Risk by Total Framingham Point Scores

Point Total	10-Year Risk
< 0	< 1%
0	1%
1	1%
2	1%
3	1%
4	1%
5	2%
6	2%
7	3%
8	4%
9	5%
10	6%
11	8%
12	10%
13	12%
14	16%
15	20%
16	25%
17 or more	≥ 30%

Estimate of 10-Year Risk for Women*

*Data in the tables that follow reproduced from National Heart, Lung, and Blood Institute (NHLBI); National Institutes of Health (NIH). (2005). NIH Publication No. 05–3290.

Framingham Point Scores by Age Group

Age	Points
20–34	−7
35–39	−3
40–44	0
45–49	3
50–54	6
55–59	8
60–64	10
65–69	12
70–74	14
75–79	16

Framingham Point Scores by Age Group and Total Cholesterol

Total Cholesterol	Age 20–39	Age 40–49	Age 50–59	Age 60–69	Age 70–79
< 160	0	0	0	0	0
160–199	4	3	2	1	1
200–239	8	6	4	2	1
240–279	11	8	5	3	2
280+	13	10	7	4	2

Framingham Point Scores by Age Group and Smoking Status

	Age 20–39	Age 40–49	Age 50–59	Age 60–69	Age 70–79
Nonsmoker	0	0	0	0	0
Smoker	9	7	4	2	1

Framingham Point Scores by HDL Level

HDL	Points
60+	−1
50–59	0
40–49	1
< 40	2

Risk Assessment Tool for Estimating Your 10-Year Risk for Having a Heart Attack

Framingham Point Scores by Systolic Blood Pressure and Treatment Status

Systolic BP	If Untreated	If Treated
< 120	0	0
120–129	1	3
130–139	2	4
140–159	3	5
160+	4	6

10-Year Risk by Total Framingham Point Scores

Point Total	10-Year Risk
< 9	< 1%
9	1%
10	1%
11	1%
12	1%
13	2%
14	2%
15	3%
16	4%
17	5%
18	6%
19	8%
20	11%
21	14%
22	17%
23	22%
24	27%
25 or more	≥ 30%

Step 3: Use your medical history, number of risk factors, and risk score to determine your risk for developing heart disease or having a heart attack in the following table.

If You Have	You Are in Category
Heart disease, diabetes, or risk score more than 20%*	I. High risk
2 or more risk factors and risk score 10–20%	II. Next highest risk
2 or more risk factors and risk score less than 10%	III. Moderate risk
0 to 1 risk factor	IV. Low-to-moderate risk

*Means that more than 20 out of 100 people in this category will have a heart attack within 10 years.

My risk category is _____.

Treating High Cholesterol

The main goal of cholesterol-lowering treatment is to lower your LDL level enough to reduce your risk for developing heart disease or having a heart attack. The higher your risk, the lower your LDL goal will be. To find your LDL goal, review the descriptions of risk categories that follow. There are two main ways to lower your cholesterol:

- Therapeutic Lifestyle Changes (TLC)—includes a cholesterol-lowering diet (called the TLC diet), physical activity, and weight management. TLC is for anyone whose LDL is above goal.

- Drug Treatment—if cholesterol-lowering drugs are needed, they are used together with TLC treatment to help lower your LDL.

If you are in . . .

- **Category I, Highest Risk,** your LDL goal is less than 100 mg/dL. You will need to begin the TLC diet to reduce your high risk even if your LDL is below 100 mg/dL. If your LDL is 100 mg/dL or above, you will need to start drug treatment at the same time as the TLC diet. If your LDL is below 100 mg/dL, you may also need to start drug treatment together with the TLC diet if your doctor finds your risk is very high (for example if you had a recent heart attack or have both heart disease and diabetes).

- **Category II, Next Highest Risk,** your LDL goal is less than 130 mg/dL. If your LDL is 130 mg/dL or above, you will need to begin treatment with the TLC diet. If your LDL is 130 mg/dL or more after 3 months on the TLC diet, you may need drug treatment along with the TLC diet. If your LDL is less than 130 mg/dL, you will need to follow the heart healthy diet for all Americans, which allows a little more saturated fat and cholesterol than the TLC diet.

- **Category III, Moderate Risk,** your LDL goal is less than 130 mg/dL. If your LDL is 130 mg/dL or above, you will need to begin the TLC diet. If your LDL is 160 mg/dL or more after you have tried the TLC diet for 3 months, you may need drug treatment along with the TLC diet. If your LDL is less than 130 mg/dL, you will need to follow the heart healthy diet for all Americans.

- **Category IV, Low-to-Moderate Risk,** your LDL goal is less than 160 mg/dL. If your LDL is 160 mg/dL or above, you will need to begin the TLC diet. If your LDL is still 160 mg/dL or more after 3 months on the TLC diet, you may need drug treatment along with the TLC diet to lower your LDL, especially if your LDL is 190 mg/dL or more. If your LDL is less than 160 mg/dL, you will need to follow the heart healthy diet for all Americans.

To reduce your risk for heart disease or keep it low, it is very important to control any other risk factors you may have, such as high blood pressure and smoking.

Lowering Cholesterol with Therapeutic Lifestyle Changes (TLC)

TLC is a set of things you can do to help lower your LDL cholesterol. The main parts of TLC are:

- *The TLC Diet.* This is a low–saturated fat, low-cholesterol eating plan that calls for less than 7 percent of calories from saturated fat and less than 200 milligrams (mg) of dietary cholesterol per day. The TLC diet recommends only enough calories to maintain a desirable weight and avoid weight gain. If your LDL is not lowered enough by reducing your saturated fat and cholesterol intakes, the amount of soluble fiber in your diet can be increased. Certain food products that contain plant stanols or plant sterols (for example, cholesterol-lowering margarines) can also be added to the TLC diet to boost its LDL-lowering power.

- *Weight Management.* Losing weight if you are overweight can help lower LDL and is especially important for those with a cluster of risk factors that includes high triglyceride and/or low HDL levels and being overweight with a large waist measurement (more than 40 inches for men and more than 35 inches for women).

- *Physical Activity.* Regular physical activity (30 minutes on most, if not all, days) is recommended for everyone. It can help raise HDL and lower LDL and is especially important for those with high triglyceride and/or low HDL levels who are overweight with a large waist measurement.

Foods low in saturated fat include fat-free or 1 percent dairy products, lean meats, fish, skinless poultry, whole-grain foods, and fruits and vegetables. Look for soft margarines (liquid or tub varieties) that are low in saturated fat and contain little or no trans fat (another type of dietary fat that can raise your cholesterol level). Limit foods high in cholesterol such as liver and other organ meats, egg yolks, and full-fat dairy products.

Good sources of soluble fiber include oats, certain fruits (such as oranges and pears) and vegetables (such as brussels sprouts and carrots), and dried peas and beans.

Drug Treatment

Even if you begin drug treatment to lower your cholesterol, you will need to continue your treatment with lifestyle changes. This will keep the dose of medicine as low as possible, and lower your risk in other ways as well. There are several types of drugs available for cholesterol lowering, including statins, bile acid sequestrants, nicotinic acid, fibric acids, and cholesterol absorption inhibitors. Your doctor can help decide which type of drug is best for you. The statin drugs are very effective in lowering LDL levels and are safe for most people. Bile acid sequestrants also lower LDL and can be used alone or in combination with statin drugs. Nicotinic acid lowers LDL and triglycerides and raises HDL. Fibric acids lower LDL somewhat but are used mainly to treat high triglyceride and low HDL levels. Cholesterol absorption inhibitors lower LDL and can be used alone or in combination with statin drugs.

Once your LDL goal has been reached, your doctor may prescribe treatment for high triglycerides and/or a low HDL level, if present. The treatment includes losing weight if needed, increasing physical activity, quitting smoking, and possibly taking a drug.

Resources

For more information about lowering cholesterol and lowering your risk for heart disease, write to the NHLBI Health Information Center, P.O. Box 30105, Bethesda, MD, 20824-0105 or call 301-592-8573.

Source: Reproduced from National Heart, Lung, and Blood Institute, National Institutes of Health (2005). NIH Publication No. 05-3290.

Name: _____ Course Number: _____

Section: _____ Date: _____

Diabetes Risk Factors

According to the National Diabetes Education Program of the National Institutes of Health and the Centers for Disease Control and Prevention, there are many factors that increase your risk for diabetes. To find out about your risk, note each item on this list that applies to you.

Directions: Next to each statement, check each item that applies to you.

Risk Factor	Yes
I am 45 years of age or older.	
The At-Risk Weight Chart shows my current weight puts me at risk. (See chart that follows)	
I have a parent, brother, or sister with diabetes.	
My family background is African American, Hispanic/Latino, American Indian, Asian American, or Pacific Islander.	
I have had diabetes while I was pregnant (this is called gestational diabetes) *or* I gave birth to a baby weighing 9 pounds or more.	
I have been told that my blood glucose (blood sugar) levels are higher than normal.	
My blood pressure is 140/90 mmHg or higher, or I have been told I have high blood pressure.	
My cholesterol (lipid) levels are not normal. My HDL cholesterol ("good cholesterol") is less than 35 mg/dL or my triglyceride level is higher than 250 mg/dL.	
I am fairly inactive. I am physically active less than three times a week.	
I have been told that I have polycystic ovary syndrome (PCOS).	
The skin around my neck or in my armpits appears dirty no matter how much I scrub it. The skin appears dark, thick, and velvety. This is called acanthosis nigricans.	
I have been told that I have blood vessel problems in my heart, brain, or legs.	

If you have any of these items, be sure to talk with your health care team about your risk for diabetes and whether you should be tested.

At-Risk Weight Chart

Find your height in the correct section of the chart. If your weight is equal to or greater than the weight listed, you are at increased risk for type 2 diabetes.

If You Are Not Asian American or Pacific Islander at Risk BMI ≥ 25	
Height	Weight
4'10"	119
4'11"	124
5'0"	128
5'1"	132
5'2"	136
5'3"	141
5'4"	145
5'5"	150
5'6"	155
5'7"	159
5'8"	164
5'9"	169
5'10"	174
5'11"	179
6'0"	184
6'1"	189
6'2"	194
6'3"	200
6'4"	205

If You Are Asian American at Risk BMI ≥ 23	
Height	Weight
4'10"	110
4'11"	114
5'0"	118
5'1"	122
5'2"	126
5'3"	130
5'4"	134
5'5"	138
5'6"	142
5'7"	146
5'8"	151
5'9"	155
5'10"	160
5'11"	165
6'0"	169
6'1"	174
6'2"	179
6'3"	184
6'4"	189

If You Are Pacific Islander at Risk BMI ≥ 26	
Height	**Weight**
4'10"	124
4'11"	128
5'0"	133
5'1"	137
5'2"	142
5'3"	146
5'4"	151
5'5"	156
5'6"	161
5'7"	166
5'8"	171
5'9"	176
5'10"	181
5'11"	186
6'0"	191
6'1"	197
6'2"	202
6'3"	208
6'4"	213

Know Your Blood Glucose Numbers

	Fasting Blood Glucose Test	**2-Hour Oral Glucose Tolerance Test**
Normal	Below 100	Below 140
Prediabetes	100–125	140–199
Diabetes	126 or above	200 or above

Source: Reproduced from National Diabetes Education Program, National Institutes of Health and the Centers for Disease Control and Prevention. (2012). Diabetes risk factors. Online: http://ndep.nih.gov/am-i-at-risk/DiabetesRiskFactors.aspx.

Name: _____ Course Number: _____

Section: _____ Date: _____

My Cardiovascular Disease Risk

Directions

1. Go to the online assessment tool "Your Disease Risk: The Source on Prevention" at http://www.yourdiseaserisk.wustl.edu. Here, you can determine your risk for developing heart disease, diabetes, and stroke in the United States and get personalized tips for preventing each disease.

2. Click on the "What is your heart disease risk?" link, and then click "Questionnaire."

3. Is your risk low, average, or high? _____

4. Click on the "What makes up your risk?" button, and then list the factors that raise your risk and the factors that lower your risk.

   Factors that raise my risk for heart disease: _____

   Factors that lower my risk for heart disease: _____

5. Click on the "What is your diabetes risk?" link, and then click "Questionnaire."

6. Is your risk low, average, or high? _____

7. Click on the "What makes up your risk?" button, and then list the factors that raise your risk and the factors that lower your risk.

   Factors that raise my risk for diabetes: _____

   Factors that lower my risk for diabetes: _____

8. Click on the "What is your stroke risk?" link, and then click "Questionnaire."

9. Is your risk low, average, or high? _____

10. Click on the "What makes up your risk?" button, and then list the factors that raise your risk and the factors that lower your risk.

    Factors that raise my risk for stroke: _____

    Factors that lower my risk for stroke: _____

Name: _____   Course Number: _____

Section: _____   Date: _____

Check Your Physical Activity and Heart Disease IQ

Directions: Test how much you know about how physical activity affects your heart. Mark each statement true or false. See how you did by checking the answers on the next page.

	True	False
1. Regular physical activity can reduce your chances of getting heart disease.	____	____
2. Most people get enough physical activity from their normal daily routine.	____	____
3. You don't have to train like a marathon runner to become more physically fit.	____	____
4. Exercise programs do not require a lot of time to be very effective.	____	____
5. People who need to lose some weight are the only ones who will benefit from regular physical activity.	____	____
6. All exercises give you the same benefits.	____	____
7. The older you are, the less active you need to be.	____	____
8. It doesn't take a lot of money or expensive equipment to become physically fit.	____	____
9. Many risks and injuries can occur with exercise.	____	____
10. You should consult a doctor before starting a physical activity program.	____	____
11. People who have had a heart attack should not start any physical activity program.	____	____
12. To help stay physically active, you should perform a variety of activities.	____	____

Answers to the Physical Activity and Heart Disease IQ Quiz

1. **True.** Heart disease is almost twice as likely to develop in inactive people. Being physically inactive is a risk factor for heart disease along with cigarette smoking, high blood pressure, high blood cholesterol, and being overweight. The more risk factors you have, the greater your chance for heart disease. Regular physical activity (even mild to moderate exercise) can reduce this risk.

2. **False.** Most Americans are very busy but not very active. Every American adult should make a habit of getting 30 minutes of low to moderate levels of physical activity daily. This includes walking, gardening, and walking up stairs. If you are inactive now, begin by doing a few minutes of activity each day. If you only do some activity every once in a while, try to work something into your routine every day.

3. **True.** Low- to moderate-intensity activities, such as pleasure walking, stair climbing, yardwork, housework, dancing, and home exercises can have both short- and long-term benefits. If you are inactive, the key is to get started. One great way is to take a walk for 10 to 15 minutes during your lunch break, or take your dog for a walk every day. At least 30 minutes of physical activity every day can help to improve your heart health.

4. **True.** It takes only a few minutes a day to become more physically active. If you don't have 30 minutes in your schedule for an exercise break, try to find two 15-minute periods or even three 10-minute periods. These exercise breaks will soon become a habit you can't live without.

5. **False.** People who are physically active experience many positive benefits. Regular physical activity gives you more energy, reduces stress, and helps you to sleep better. It helps to lower high blood pressure and improves blood cholesterol levels. Physical activity helps to tone your muscles, burns off calories to help you lose extra pounds or stay at your desirable weight, and helps control your appetite. It can also increase muscle strength, help your heart and lungs work more efficiently, and let you enjoy your life more fully.

6. **False.** Low-intensity activities—if performed daily—can have some long-term health benefits and can lower your risk of heart disease. Regular, brisk, and sustained exercise for at least 30 minutes, three to four times a week, such as brisk walking, jogging, or swimming, is necessary to improve the efficiency of your heart and lungs and burn off extra calories. These activities are called aerobic—meaning the body uses oxygen to produce the energy needed for the activity. Other activities, depending on the type, may give you other benefits such as increased flexibility or muscle strength.

7. **False.** Although we tend to become less active with age, physical activity is still important. In fact, regular physical activity in older persons increases their capacity to do everyday activities. In general, middle-aged and older people benefit from regular physical activity just as young people do. What is important, at any age, is tailoring the activity program to your own fitness level.

8. **True.** Many activities require little or no equipment. For example, brisk walking only requires a comfortable pair of walking shoes. Many communities offer free or inexpensive recreation facilities and physical activity classes. Check your shopping

malls because many of them are open early and late for people who do not wish to walk alone, in the dark, or in bad weather.

9. **False.** The most common risk in exercising is injury to the muscles and joints. Such injuries are usually caused by exercising too hard for too long, particularly if a person has been inactive. To avoid injuries, try to build up your level of activity gradually, listen to your body for warning pains, be aware of possible signs of heart problems (such as pain or pressure in the left or midchest area, left neck, shoulder, or arm during or just after exercising, or sudden light-headedness, cold sweat, pallor, or fainting), and be prepared for special weather conditions.

10. **True.** You should ask your doctor before you start (or greatly increase) your physical activity if you have a medical condition such as high blood pressure, have pains or pressure in the chest and shoulder, feel dizzy or faint, get breathless after mild exertion, are middle-aged or older and have not been physically active, or plan a vigorous activity program. If none of these apply, start slow and get moving.

11. **False.** Regular physical activity can help reduce your risk of having another heart attack. People who include regular physical activity in their lives after a heart attack improve their chances of survival and can improve how they feel and look. If you have had a heart attack, consult your doctor to be sure you are following a safe and effective exercise program that will help prevent heart pain and further damage from overexertion.

12. **True.** Pick several different activities that you like doing. You will be more likely to stay with it. Plan short-term and long-term goals. Keep a record of your progress, and check it regularly to see the progress you have made. Get your family and friends to join in. They can help keep you going.

Source: Reproduced from National Heart, Lung, and Blood Institute (NHLBI) and National Institutes of Health (NIH). (1996, August). *Physical Activity & Heart Disease IQ* (NIH Pub. No. 96-3795). Online: http://www.nhlbi.nih.gov/health/public/heart/obesity/phy_act.htm.

Chapter 14: Critical Thinking Questions

Protecting Your Cardiovascular System

1. Make a list of all the six major modifiable risk factors that increase your chances of getting CVD. Which risk factors pertain to you? How can you modify or change any of these risk factors?

2. A risk factor of cardiovascular disease is family history. Family history of CVD does not guarantee that you will get the disease, and neither does it cancel out the importance of a healthy lifestyle. A family history of CVD does predispose you to the disease, so it is important for you to determine your family CVD history. Construct a family tree by listing your biological parents, siblings, grandparents (maternal and paternal), and aunts and uncles (maternal and paternal). Next to each name, list the CVD disease and the age at which it was discovered. Your family may be helpful with this activity. After completing your tree, you may want to share it with your family and discuss prevention efforts.

3. Elena is a 21-year-old college student who is very studious. Because her studies are her number one priority (she wants to go to graduate school), Elena finds it difficult to make time to maintain a healthy lifestyle, despite knowing how important it is. Although Elena is not a regular smoker, she has a tendency to smoke when under stress (studying for finals) and frequently eats nonnutritious snacks. Elena was active in high school sports, but she does not seem to find time for sports now that she is in college. As a matter of fact, she has gained about 15 pounds, although she would not be considered overweight. What can you suggest to help Elena reduce her risk of cardiovascular disease?

_____

_____

_____

_____

_____

_____

_____

_____

_____

_____

_____

Critical Thinking Questions

Name: ——————————————————————— Course Number: ———————————

Section: ——————————————————————— Date: ———————————————

Reducing Your Cancer Risk

The following 20 descriptions of individual choices are based on the 2012 American Cancer Society's *Guidelines on Nutrition and Physical Activity for Cancer Prevention.*

Part I. For each statement, check the column that best describes you. Please answer each statement as you currently are (rather than how you think you should be).

Healthy Choices for Cancer Prevention	Never or Rarely	Sometimes	Usually or Always
1. I am as lean as possible and have been throughout my life without being underweight.			
2. I have avoided excess weight gain at all ages.			
3. I get regular physical activity and limit intake of high-calorie foods and drinks to help maintain a healthy weight.			
4. I get at least 150 minutes of moderate-intensity or 75 minutes of vigorous-intensity activity each week (or a combination of these), preferably spread throughout the week.			
5. I limit sedentary behavior such as sitting, lying down, and watching TV and other forms of screen-based entertainment.			
6. I read food labels and am aware of portion sizes and calories. I know that "low-fat" or "non-fat" does not necessarily mean "low-calorie."			
7. I eat smaller portions when eating high-calorie foods.			
8. I choose vegetables, whole fruit, and other low-calorie foods instead of calorie-dense foods such as French fries, potato and other chips, ice cream, donuts, and other sweets.			
9. I limit my intake of sugar-sweetened beverages such as soft drinks, sports drinks, and fruit-flavored drinks.			
10. When I eat away from home, I'm especially mindful to choose foods low in calories, fat, and added sugar, and I avoid eating large portion sizes.			

11. I limit my intake of processed meats such as bacon, sausage, lunch meats, and hot dogs.			
12. I choose fish, poultry, or beans instead of red meat (beef, pork, and lamb).			
13. If I eat red meat, I choose lean cuts and eat smaller portions.			
14. I prepare meat, poultry, and fish by baking, broiling, or poaching rather than by frying or charbroiling.			
15. I include vegetables and fruits at every meal and for snacks.			
16. I eat a variety of vegetables and fruits each day.			
17. I choose whole fruits and vegetables; I choose 100% juice if I drink vegetable or fruit juices.			
18. I limit my use of creamy sauces, dressings, and dips with fruits and vegetables.			
19. I choose whole-grain breads, pasta, and cereals (such as barley and oats) instead of breads, cereals, and pasta made from refined grains, and brown rice instead of white rice.			
20. I limit my intake of refined-carbohydrate foods, including pastries, candy, sugar-sweetened breakfast cereals, and other high-sugar foods.			
Totals			

Source: Data from American Cancer Society. (2012). *ACS Guidelines on Nutrition and Physical Activity for Cancer Prevention.* Online: http://www.cancer.org/Healthy/EatHealthyGetActive/ACSGuidelinesonNutritionPhysical ActivityforCancerPrevention/index.

Part II. Select one behavior that you checked "never or rarely" or "sometimes" that you plan to work on in the next 30 days to begin reducing your cancer risk.

Target behavior: _____

Step 1: Your goal is to commit to this target behavior soon. You will do so by setting small, realistic goals and creating a plan to take action.

What changes will you need to make to achieve this target behavior? In other words, what will you need to do differently to succeed?

_____

_____

Write one or two SMART goals that will help you achieve this target behavior:

1. _____

2. _____

Commit to take action. Set a start date: _____

Tell someone what you plan to do. Being accountable to others motivates you and also offers you support and encouragement.

Who did you tell? _____

Signature: _____

Step 2: Your goal is to firmly establish this behavior as a lifelong habit by anticipating problems and preparing to overcome failures, and by rewarding your success to stay committed.

Track your progress. For 7 days after your start date, keep track of the results of trying to meet your SMART goal(s).
Evaluate your progress and continue or modify your plan:

Smart Goals	Dates	Results

_____

_____

In what ways have you benefited from adopting this behavior?

_____

_____

What motivates you the most to continue practicing this behavior and why?

_____

_____

Reward your progress. Permanently changing lifestyle behaviors takes patience and consistent positive reinforcement. List several rewards you could give yourself for meeting your goals:

_____

_____

Select a reward for meeting your goal(s) for 7 days: _____

Select a reward for meeting your goal(s) for 1 month: _____

Name: _____ Course Number: _____

Section: _____ Date: _____

My Cancer Risk

Directions

1. Go to the online assessment tool "Your Disease Risk: The Source on Prevention" at http://www.yourdiseaserisk.wustl.edu. Here, you can find out your risk of developing cancer in the United States and get personalized tips for preventing cancer.

2. Click on "What Is Your Cancer Risk?" and choose three different cancers (bladder, breast, cervical, colon, kidney, lung, melanoma, ovarian, pancreatic, prostate, stomach, uterine) and assess risk by completing the accompanying questionnaire.

3. Is your risk low, average, or high for _____ cancer? _____

4. Click on "What makes up your risk?" and list the factors that raise your risk and the factors that lower your risk.

   Factors that raise my risk of _____ cancer: _____

   Factors that lower my risk of _____ cancer: _____

5. Is your risk low, average, or high for _____ cancer? _____

6. Click on "What makes up your risk?" and list the factors that raise your risk and the factors that lower your risk.

   Factors that raise my risk of _____ cancer: _____

   Factors that lower my risk of _____ cancer: _____

7. Is your risk low, average, or high for _____ cancer? _____

8. Click on "What makes up your risk?" and list the factors that raise your risk and the factors that lower your risk.

   Factors that raise my risk of _____ cancer: _____

   Factors that lower my risk of_____ cancer: _____

Chapter 15: Critical Thinking Questions

Reducing Your Cancer Risk

1. Make a list of all the modifiable risk factors that increase your chance of getting cancer. Order the list from the highest to lowest risk. Which risk factors pertain to you? How can you modify or change these risk factors?

2. Family history is a risk factor for cancer. A family history of cancer does not guarantee that you will get the disease, and neither does it cancel out the importance of a healthy lifestyle (not smoking, good dietary habits, and regular physical activity). A family history of cancer does predispose you to the disease; therefore, it is important for you to determine your family cancer history. Construct a family tree by listing your biological parents, siblings, grandparents (maternal and paternal), and aunts and uncles (maternal and paternal). A sample family cancer history diagram is shown here. Next to each name, list the type of cancer and the age at which it was discovered. Your family may be helpful with this activity. After completing your tree, you may want to share it with your family and discuss prevention efforts (include cancer screenings and early detection methods).

3. Do you have any family members or friends like Katrina who would like to quit smoking? If yes, go online to the American Cancer Society website and search for ways to quit smoking. After completing this activity, sit down and share the information with the individual trying to quit smoking.

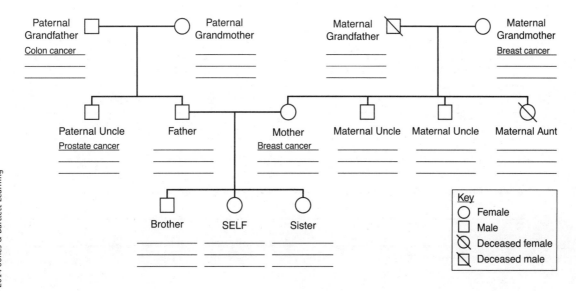

Critical Thinking Questions

Name: _____   Course Number: _____

Section: _____   Date: _____

STI Quiz

Test Your STI Knowledge

1. You can get several sexually transmitted infections at one time.

   True or False?

2. Most sexually transmitted infections can be treated and cured without medical attention.

   True or False?

3. If the signs of a sexually transmitted infection go away, you are cured.

   True or False?

4. If you use birth control pills, you can get a sexually transmitted infection.

   True or False?

5. You always know when you have a sexually transmitted infection.

   True or False?

6. People who get a sexually transmitted infection have a lot of sex partners.

   True or False?

7. All types of sexually transmitted infections can be cured.

   True or False?

8. Parental consent is needed before you are treated for a sexually transmitted infection if you are under 18 years of age.

   True or False?

9. You can have no symptoms yet be infected with a sexually transmitted infection and be able to pass it on to someone else.

   True or False?

10. You can wash away a sexually transmitted infection.

    True or False?

11. All genital infections are a result of sexual contact.

    True or False?

12. You can get a sexually transmitted infection more than once.

True or False?

13. More than 15 million new cases of sexually transmitted infections are diagnosed each year in the United States.

True or False?

14. One in 10 people in the United States have a sexually transmitted infection.

True or False?

Answers to STI Quiz

1. You can get several sexually transmitted infections at one time.

TRUE. It is possible to have many STIs at one time. In fact, having one STI may make it more likely that a person will acquire more STIs. For example, the open sores from herpes create a place for HIV to be transmitted.

2. Most sexually transmitted infections can be treated and cured without medical attention.

FALSE. You can NOT cure yourself of an STI. Only a health practitioner can correctly diagnose and treat you.

3. If the signs of a sexually transmitted infection go away, you are cured.

FALSE. The symptoms may go away, but your body is still infected. For example, syphilis is characterized by three stages. In the first stage, a painless sore called a chancre appears for about a week and then goes away.

4. If you use birth control pills, you can get a sexually transmitted infection.

TRUE. Birth control pills do not protect you from STI infection. The only method of birth control that can help reduce the risk of getting an STI is condoms.

5. You always know when you have a sexually transmitted infection.

FALSE. Not all STIs have detectable symptoms. You may feel fine, have no unusual odors, look healthy, and still be infected with an STI. For example, 75 percent of women and 50 percent of men have no symptoms when infected with chlamydia.

6. People who get a sexually transmitted infection have a lot of sex partners.

FALSE. It only takes one time if a person is having sex with an infected partner to get an STI.

7. All types of sexually transmitted infections can be cured.

FALSE. Some STIs are viruses and therefore cannot be cured. There is no cure presently for herpes, HIV/AIDS, or genital warts. Some STIs are treatable (to lessen pain and irritation with symptoms) but not curable.

8. Parental consent is needed before you are treated for a sexually transmitted infection if you are under 18 years of age.

FALSE. You can receive confidential treatment for an STI if you are age 12 or over. Your parents do not have to be notified.

9. You can have no symptoms yet be infected with a sexually transmitted infection and be able to pass it on to someone else.

TRUE. A person does not always have to be experiencing symptoms to transmit an STI to a partner.

10. You can wash away a sexually transmitted infection.

FALSE. No amount of washing can make an STI go away. STIs must be diagnosed and treated by a health care provider.

11. All genital infections are a result of sexual contact.

FALSE. Some infections occur naturally, without sexual contact. Some types of vaginal infections (e.g., yeast infections) are not sexually transmitted and are due to other causes.

12. You can get a sexually transmitted infection more than once.

TRUE. Experiencing one infection with an STI does NOT mean that you can never be infected again. A person can be reinfected many times with the same STI. This is especially true if a person does not get treated for the STI and thus keeps reinfecting his/her partner with the same STI.

13. More than 15 million new cases of sexually transmitted infections are diagnosed each year in the United States.

TRUE. (CDC. www.cdc.gov/nchstp/dstd/Stats_Trends/STD_Trends.pdf)

14. One in 10 people in the United States have a sexually transmitted infection.

FALSE. One in FIVE people in the United States have a sexually transmitted infection. (ASHA. www.ashastd.org/stdfaqs/statistics.html).

Source: Reproduced from Jefferson County Public Health, Golden, Colorado. STD Quiz. Reprinted with permission. Online: http://jeffco.us/health/health_T111_R70.htm.

Name: _____ Course Number: _____

Section: _____ Date: _____

An Ounce of Prevention

Conduct an informal interview of students (not from this class) regarding their feelings about the pros and cons of the following STI safer sex techniques for college students.

	Pros	Cons
Abstinence		
Delaying having sex with a potential partner until you know him/her well enough to assess risk and discuss STI concerns		
Long-term monogamous sexual relationship with an uninfected partner		
Using a latex condom, dental dam, female condom, or other barrier while performing sexual acts		
Limiting the number of concurrent sexual partners		
Refraining from the use of alcohol and other drugs before having sex		

Based on the information you have gathered from your peers, what do you recommend as an effective strategy for college students to reduce the risk of contracting sexually transmitted infections? Why?

_____

_____

_____

_____

Name: ———————————————————————— Course Number: ————————————

Section: ———————————————————————— Date: ————————————————

Can You Be Assertive When You Need to Be?

To take the necessary actions to prevent contracting a sexually transmitted infection, you will have to be assertive. That is, you will need to resist pressure to engage in sexual activity if you choose not to, and you will need to insist on the use of a condom and other safer-sex precautions if you do decide to engage in sex. Do you have assertiveness skills? To find out, write an assertive response to each of the following situations.

1. You are on a date and your partner insists on engaging in a sexual activity that you decide is not for you at that time. You say:

———

———

———

———

2. Your partner argues that condoms diminish the sensation. You respond by saying:

———

———

———

———

3. Your partner states that she or he has been tested for STIs and the test was negative. Therefore, there are no reasons for using safer-sex techniques. You respond by saying:

———

———

———

———

To Be Assertive, You Need To

- Specify the behavior or situation to which the statement refers.

- Relate your feelings about that situation.

- Suggest a remedy or what you would prefer to see occur.

- Identify the consequences of the change; what will happen if it occurs and what will happen if it does not occur.

  Now, check your responses and revise them to be consistent with these assertiveness principles.

Source: Reproduced from J.S. Greenberg, C.E. Bruess, & S. Conklin. (2007). *Exploring the Dimensions of Human Sexuality*, 3rd ed. Sudbury, MA: Jones & Bartlett, 604–605.

Name: ———————————————————— Course Number: ——————————

Section: ———————————————————— Date: ——————————

Chapter 16: Critical Thinking Questions

Preventing Sexually Transmitted Infections

1. Jeremy and Christina have chosen to abstain from sexual intercourse. Describe for yourself the pros and cons of sexual abstinence. Have you been able to discuss your thoughts about sexuality with your current partner?

2. As more and more people become infected with HIV, more students attending universities and colleges are infected with HIV. Many universities have residence halls with living quarters that accommodate two to four people of the same gender. Is it necessary for universities to notify students in a residence hall if a person living there is HIV-positive? If not, why not?

3. Herpes is a sexually transmitted infection that lasts a lifetime; however, herpes can be managed with medication. Explain, in detail, how you would go about telling your new partner that you have herpes.

4. You and your best college friend are talking, and your friend confides to you that about 2 months ago he may have had sexual intercourse with someone who could be HIV-positive, but your friend is not having any symptoms. What advice would you give him?

———————————————————————————————————————
———————————————————————————————————————
———————————————————————————————————————
———————————————————————————————————————
———————————————————————————————————————
———————————————————————————————————————
———————————————————————————————————————
———————————————————————————————————————
———————————————————————————————————————
———————————————————————————————————————
———————————————————————————————————————
———————————————————————————————————————

© 2014 Jones & Bartlett Learning

Critical Thinking Questions

Name: ——————————————————————— Course Number: ———————————————

Section: ——————————————————————— Date: ———————————————

Diet and Activity Records

The diet and activity records in this appendix provide enough forms to record your intakes and expenditures for an entire week. The forms for each day are placed together. Use as many forms as necessary to complete your assigment.

Diet Record Day 1

Name: _____ Date: _____

☐ Weekday
☐ Weekend Day

Eating Behavior Diary

Time of Day	M, S, or B[1]	H[2] (0–3)	Location	Activity While Eating	Others Present	Time Spent Eating	Food Eaten and Quantity (describe preparation, variety, etc., as needed)	Reason for Choice[3]	Helpings (0, –, +)[4]	S[5] (0–3)

[1] Indicate whether the eating/drinking event was a meal, a snack, or a beverage.

[2] Degree of hunger: 0 = not at all hungry; 1 = slightly hungry; 2 = moderately hungry; 3 = very hungry. If only a beverage was consumed, apply the scale to the degree of thirst.

[3] Reason for food choice: Examples include taste, habit, convenience, health, weight control, hunger, thirst, stress, comfort, offered to me, and so on.

[4] Helpings: 0 = ate all that you were first served but not more; – = ate less than what you were served; + = ate more than you were originally served.

[5] Degree of satiation: 0 = not at all satisfied; 1 = still a little hungry; 2 = satisfied and comfortable; 3 = very full.

Eating Behavior Diary

Time of Day	M, S, or B[1]	H[2] (0–3)	Location	Activity While Eating	Others Present	Time Spent Eating	Food Eaten and Quantity (describe preparation, variety, etc., as needed)	Reason for Choice[3]	Helpings (0,−,+)[4]	S[5] (0–3)

[1] Indicate whether the eating/drinking event was a meal, a snack, or a beverage.

[2] Degree of hunger: 0 = not at all hungry; 1 = slightly hungry; 2 = moderately hungry; 3 = very hungry. If only a beverage was consumed, apply the scale to the degree of thirst.

[3] Reason for food choice: Examples include taste, habit, convenience, health, weight control, hunger, thirst, stress, comfort, offered to me, and so on.

[4] Helpings: 0 = ate all that you were first served but not more; − = ate less than what you were served; + = ate more than you were originally served.

[5] Degree of satiation: 0 = not at all satisfied; 1 = still a little hungry; 2 = satisfied and comfortable; 3 = very full.

Diet and Activity Records   227

Activity Record Day 1

Name: _____ Date: _____

☐ Weekday
☐ Weekend Day

Activity Record

Time of Day	Duration (Minutes)	Description of Activity	Level of Activity

	Activity Record		
Time of Day	Duration (Minutes)	Description of Activity	Level of Activity

Total Duration: _____ (must equal 1440 minutes for the entire 24-hour period)

Diet Record Day 2

Name: _____   Date: _____

☐ Weekday
☐ Weekend Day

Eating Behavior Diary

Time of Day	M, S, or B[1]	H[2] (0–3)	Location	Activity While Eating	Others Present	Time Spent Eating	Food Eaten and Quantity (describe preparation, variety, etc., as needed)	Reason for Choice[3]	Helpings (0,−,+)[4]	S[5] (0–3)

[1] Indicate whether the eating/drinking event was a meal, a snack, or a beverage.

[2] Degree of hunger: 0 = not at all hungry; 1 = slightly hungry; 2 = moderately hungry; 3 = very hungry. If only a beverage was consumed, apply the scale to the degree of thirst.

[3] Reason for food choice: Examples include taste, habit, convenience, health, weight control, hunger, thirst, stress, comfort, offered to me, and so on.

[4] Helpings: 0 = ate all that you were first served but not more; − = ate less than what you were served; + = ate more than you were originally served.

[5] Degree of satiation: 0 = not at all satisfied; 1 = still a little hungry; 2 = satisfied and comfortable; 3 = very full.

Eating Behavior Diary

Time of Day	M, S, or B[1]	H[2] (0–3)	Location	Activity While Eating	Others Present	Time Spent Eating	Food Eaten and Quantity (describe preparation, variety, etc., as needed)	Reason for Choice[3]	Helpings (0,−,+)[4]	S[5] (0–3)

[1] Indicate whether the eating/drinking event was a meal, a snack, or a beverage.

[2] Degree of hunger: 0 = not at all hungry; 1 = slightly hungry; 2 = moderately hungry; 3 = very hungry. If only a beverage was consumed, apply the scale to the degree of thirst.

[3] Reason for food choice: Examples include taste, habit, convenience, health, weight control, hunger, thirst, stress, comfort, offered to me, and so on.

[4] Helpings: 0 = ate all that you were first served but not more; − = ate less than what you were served; + = ate more than you were originally served.

[5] Degree of satiation: 0 = not at all satisfied; 1 = still a little hungry; 2 = satisfied and comfortable; 3 = very full.

Activity Record Day 2

Name: _____ Date: _____

☐ Weekday
☐ Weekend Day

Activity Record			
Time of Day	Duration (Minutes)	Description of Activity	Level of Activity

Activity Record			
Time of Day	Duration (Minutes)	Description of Activity	Level of Activity

Total Duration: _____ (must equal 1440 minutes for the entire 24-hour period)

Diet Record Day 3

Name: _____ Date: _____

☐ Weekday
☐ Weekend Day

Eating Behavior Diary

Time of Day	M, S, or B[1]	H[2] (0–3)	Location	Activity While Eating	Others Present	Time Spent Eating	Food Eaten and Quantity (describe preparation, variety, etc. as needed)	Reason for Choice[3]	Helpings (0,−,+)[4]	S[5] (0–3)

[1] Indicate whether the eating/drinking event was a meal, a snack, or a beverage.

[2] Degree of hunger: 0 = not at all hungry; 1 = slightly hungry; 2 = moderately hungry; 3 = very hungry. If only a beverage was consumed, apply the scale to the degree of thirst.

[3] Reason for food choice: Examples include taste, habit, convenience, health, weight control, hunger, thirst, stress, comfort, offered to me, and so on.

[4] Helpings: 0 = ate all that you were first served but not more; − = ate less than what you were served; + = ate more than you were originally served.

[5] Degree of satiation: 0 = not at all satisfied; 1 = still a little hungry; 2 = satisfied and comfortable; 3 = very full.

Eating Behavior Diary

Time of Day	M, S, or B[1]	H[2] (0–3)	Location	Activity While Eating	Others Present	Time Spent Eating	Food Eaten and Quantity (describe preparation, variety, etc., as needed)	Reason for Choice[3]	Helpings (0,–,+)[4]	S[5] (0–3)

[1] Indicate whether the eating/drinking event was a meal, a snack, or a beverage.

[2] Degree of hunger: 0 = not at all hungry; 1 = slightly hungry; 2 = moderately hungry; 3 = very hungry. If only a beverage was consumed, apply the scale to the degree of thirst.

[3] Reason for food choice: Examples include taste, habit, convenience, health, weight control, hunger, thirst, stress, comfort, offered to me, and so on.

[4] Helpings: 0 = ate all that you were first served but not more; – = ate less than what you were served; + = ate more than you were originally served.

[5] Degree of satiation: 0 = not at all satisfied; 1 = still a little hungry; 2 = satisfied and comfortable; 3 = very full.

Activity Record Day 3

Name: _____   Date: _____   ☐ Weekday
                                                             ☐ Weekend Day

Activity Record			
Time of Day	Duration (Minutes)	Description of Activity	Level of Activity

	Activity Record		
Time of Day	Duration (Minutes)	Description of Activity	Level of Activity

Total Duration: _____ (must equal 1440 minutes for the entire 24-hour period)

Diet Record Day 4

Name: _____   Date: _____   ☐ Weekday
☐ Weekend Day

Eating Behavior Diary

Time of Day	M, S, or B[1]	H[2] (0–3)	Location	Activity While Eating	Others Present	Time Spent Eating	Food Eaten and Quantity (describe preparation, variety, etc., as needed)	Reason for Choice[3]	Helpings (0,−,+)[4]	S[5] (0–3)

[1] Indicate whether the eating/drinking event was a meal, a snack, or a beverage.

[2] Degree of hunger: 0 = not at all hungry; 1 = slightly hungry; 2 = moderately hungry; 3 = very hungry. If only a beverage was consumed, apply the scale to the degree of thirst.

[3] Reason for food choice: Examples include taste, habit, convenience, health, weight control, hunger, thirst, stress, comfort, offered to me, and so on.

[4] Helpings: 0 = ate all that you were first served but not more; − = ate less than what you were served; + = ate more than you were originally served.

[5] Degree of satiation: 0 = not at all satisfied; 1 = still a little hungry; 2 = satisfied and comfortable; 3 = very full.

Eating Behavior Diary

Time of Day	M, S, or B[1]	H[2] (0–3)	Location	Activity While Eating	Others Present	Time Spent Eating	Food Eaten and Quantity (describe preparation, variety, etc., as needed)	Reason for Choice[3]	Helpings (0,–,+)[4]	S[5] (0–3)

[1] Indicate whether the eating/drinking event was a meal, a snack, or a beverage.

[2] Degree of hunger: 0 = not at all hungry; 1 = slightly hungry; 2 = moderately hungry; 3 = very hungry. If only a beverage was consumed, apply the scale to the degree of thirst.

[3] Reason for food choice: Examples include taste, habit, convenience, health, weight control, hunger, thirst, stress, comfort, offered to me, and so on.

[4] Helpings: 0 = ate all that you were first served but not more; – = ate less than what you were served; + = ate more than you were originally served.

[5] Degree of satiation: 0 = not at all satisfied; 1 = still a little hungry; 2 = satisfied and comfortable; 3 = very full.

Diet and Activity Records

Activity Record Day 4

Name: _____   Date: _____   ☐ Weekday
☐ Weekend Day

Activity Record

Time of Day	Duration (Minutes)	Description of Activity	Level of Activity

	Activity Record		
Time of Day	Duration (Minutes)	Description of Activity	Level of Activity

Total Duration: _____ (must equal 1440 minutes for the entire 24-hour period)

Diet Record Day 5

Name: _____ Date: _____

☐ Weekday
☐ Weekend Day

Eating Behavior Diary

Time of Day	M, S, or B[1]	H[2] (0–3)	Location	Activity While Eating	Others Present	Time Spent Eating	Food Eaten and Quantity (describe preparation, variety, etc., as needed)	Reason for Choice[3]	Helpings (0,−,+)[4]	S[5] (0–3)

[1] Indicate whether the eating/drinking event was a meal, a snack, or a beverage.
[2] Degree of hunger: 0 = not at all hungry; 1 = slightly hungry; 2 = moderately hungry; 3 = very hungry. If only a beverage was consumed, apply the scale to the degree of thirst.
[3] Reason for food choice: Examples include taste, habit, convenience, health, weight control, hunger, thirst, stress, comfort, offered to me, and so on.
[4] Helpings: 0 = ate all that you were first served but not more; − = ate less than what you were served; + = ate more than you were originally served.
[5] Degree of satiation: 0 = not at all satisfied; 1 = still a little hungry; 2 = satisfied and comfortable; 3 = very full.

Eating Behavior Diary

Time of Day	M, S, or B[1]	H[2] (0–3)	Location	Activity While Eating	Others Present	Time Spent Eating	Food Eaten and Quantity (describe preparation, variety, etc., as needed)	Reason for Choice[3]	Helpings (0,−,+)[4]	S[5] (0–3)

[1] Indicate whether the eating/drinking event was a meal, a snack, or a beverage.

[2] Degree of hunger: 0 = not at all hungry; 1 = slightly hungry; 2 = moderately hungry; 3 = very hungry. If only a beverage was consumed, apply the scale to the degree of thirst.

[3] Reason for food choice: Examples include taste, habit, convenience, health, weight control, hunger, thirst, stress, comfort, offered to me, and so on.

[4] Helpings: 0 = ate all that you were first served but not more; − = ate less than what you were served; + = ate more than you were originally served.

[5] Degree of satiation: 0 = not at all satisfied; 1 = still a little hungry; 2 = satisfied and comfortable; 3 = very full.

Activity Record Day 5

Name: _____   Date: _____

☐ Weekday
☐ Weekend Day

Activity Record

Time of Day	Duration (Minutes)	Description of Activity	Level of Activity

	Activity Record		
Time of Day	Duration (Minutes)	Description of Activity	Level of Activity

Total Duration: _____ (must equal 1440 minutes for the entire 24-hour period)

Diet Record Day 6

Name: _____ Date: _____ ☐ Weekday ☐ Weekend Day

Eating Behavior Diary

Time of Day	M, S, or B[1]	H[2] (0–3)	Location	Activity While Eating	Others Present	Time Spent Eating	Food Eaten and Quantity (describe preparation, variety, etc., as needed)	Reason for Choice[3]	Helpings (0,–,+)[4]	S[5] (0–3)

[1] Indicate whether the eating/drinking event was a meal, a snack, or a beverage.

[2] Degree of hunger: 0 = not at all hungry; 1 = slightly hungry; 2 = moderately hungry; 3 = very hungry. If only a beverage was consumed, apply the scale to the degree of thirst.

[3] Reason for food choice: Examples include taste, habit, convenience, health, weight control, hunger, thirst, stress, comfort, offered to me, and so on.

[4] Helpings: 0 = ate all that you were first served but not more; – = ate less than what you were served; + = ate more than you were originally served.

[5] Degree of satiation: 0 = not at all satisfied; 1 = still a little hungry; 2 = satisfied and comfortable; 3 = very full.

Eating Behavior Diary

Time of Day	M, S, or B[1]	H[2] (0–3)	Location	Activity While Eating	Others Present	Time Spent Eating	Food Eaten and Quantity (describe preparation, variety, etc., as needed)	Reason for Choice[3]	Helpings (0,−,+)[4]	S[5] (0–3)

[1] Indicate whether the eating/drinking event was a meal, a snack, or a beverage.

[2] Degree of hunger: 0 = not at all hungry; 1 = slightly hungry; 2 = moderately hungry; 3 = very hungry. If only a beverage was consumed, apply the scale to the degree of thirst.

[3] Reason for food choice: Examples include taste, habit, convenience, health, weight control, hunger, thirst, stress, comfort, offered to me, and so on.

[4] Helpings: 0 = ate all that you were first served but not more; − = ate less than what you were served; + = ate more than you were originally served.

[5] Degree of satiation: 0 = not at all satisfied; 1 = still a little hungry; 2 = satisfied and comfortable; 3 = very full.

Activity Record Day 6

Name: _____ Date: _____

☐ Weekday
☐ Weekend Day

Activity Record

Time of Day	Duration (Minutes)	Description of Activity	Level of Activity

Activity Record			
Time of Day	Duration (Minutes)	Description of Activity	Level of Activity

Total Duration: _____ (must equal 1440 minutes for the entire 24-hour period)

Diet Record Day 7

Name: _____   Date: _____

☐ Weekday
☐ Weekend Day

Eating Behavior Diary

Time of Day	M, S, or B[1]	H[2] (0–3)	Location	Activity While Eating	Others Present	Time Spent Eating	Food Eaten and Quantity (describe preparation, variety, etc., as needed)	Reason for Choice[3]	Helpings (0, –, +)[4]	S[5] (0–3)

[1] Indicate whether the eating/drinking event was a meal, a snack, or a beverage.
[2] Degree of hunger: 0 = not at all hungry; 1 = slightly hungry; 2 = moderately hungry; 3 = very hungry. If only a beverage was consumed, apply the scale to the degree of thirst.
[3] Reason for food choice: Examples include taste, habit, convenience, health, weight control, hunger, thirst, stress, comfort, offered to me, and so on.
[4] Helpings: 0 = ate all that you were first served but not more; – = ate less than what you were served; + = ate more than you were originally served.
[5] Degree of satiation: 0 = not at all satisfied; 1 = still a little hungry; 2 = satisfied and comfortable; 3 = very full.

Eating Behavior Diary

Time of Day	M, S, or B[1]	H[2] (0–3)	Location	Activity While Eating	Others Present	Time Spent Eating	Food Eaten and Quantity (describe preparation, variety, etc., as needed)	Reason for Choice[3]	Helpings (0,−,+)[4]	S[5] (0–3)

[1] Indicate whether the eating/drinking event was a meal, a snack, or a beverage.

[2] Degree of hunger: 0 = not at all hungry; 1 = slightly hungry; 2 = moderately hungry; 3 = very hungry. If only a beverage was consumed, apply the scale to the degree of thirst.

[3] Reason for food choice: Examples include taste, habit, convenience, health, weight control, hunger, thirst, stress, comfort, offered to me, and so on.

[4] Helpings: 0 = ate all that you were first served but not more; − = ate less than what you were served; + = ate more than you were originally served.

[5] Degree of satiation: 0 = not at all satisfied; 1 = still a little hungry; 2 = satisfied and comfortable; 3 = very full.

Activity Record Day 7

Name: _____   Date: _____

☐ Weekday
☐ Weekend Day

Activity Record

Time of Day	Duration (Minutes)	Description of Activity	Level of Activity

Activity Record			
Time of Day	Duration (Minutes)	Description of Activity	Level of Activity

Total Duration: _____ (must equal 1440 minutes for the entire 24-hour period)

Name: _____ Course Number: _____

Section: _____ Date: _____

Growth Charts: Stature-for-Age and Weight-for-Age Percentiles for Children and Teenagers

For children and teenagers, healthy weight status is defined differently than it is for adults. Because children and teenagers are still growing, boys and girls develop at different rates. The body mass index (BMI) for a child aged 2 to 20 years is determined by comparing his or her weight and height against the appropriate growth chart that accounts for age and gender. (See the Centers for Disease Control and Prevention's [CDC] growth charts for boys and girls on the following pages.)

Tracking Changes in BMI-for-Age

1. Select the appropriate chart.

2. Calculate BMI using the formula on the growth chart or using the online BMI percentile calculator available at http://apps.nccd.cdc.gov/dnpabmi/Calculator.aspx.

3. Plot the BMI percentile number obtained from the formula or calculator against the child's age.

4. Use the following table to interpret the results.

BMI Percentile-for-Age	Suggests the Child/Teenager Is
At or over the 95th percentile	Obese
Between the 85th and 95th percentiles	Overweight
Between 15th and 85th percentiles	Probably at a healthy weight
Between 5th and 15th percentiles	Possibly at risk for underweight
Under the 5th percentile	Underweight

5. Every few months, recalculate the child's or teen's BMI percentile and plot on the chart.

2 to 20 years: Boys
Stature-for-Age and Weight-for-Age Percentiles

NAME _____

RECORD # _____

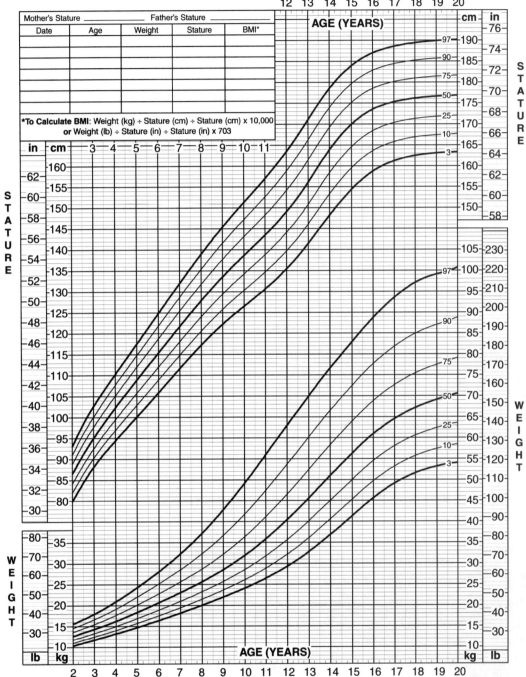

Source: Developed by the National Center for Health Statistics in collaboration with the National Center for Chronic Disease Prevention and Health Promotion (2000). Online: http://www.cdc.gov/growthcharts.

Growth Charts: Stature-for-Age and Weight-for-Age Percentiles for Children and Teenagers

2 to 20 years: Girls
Stature-for-Age and Weight-for-Age Percentiles

NAME _____

RECORD # _____

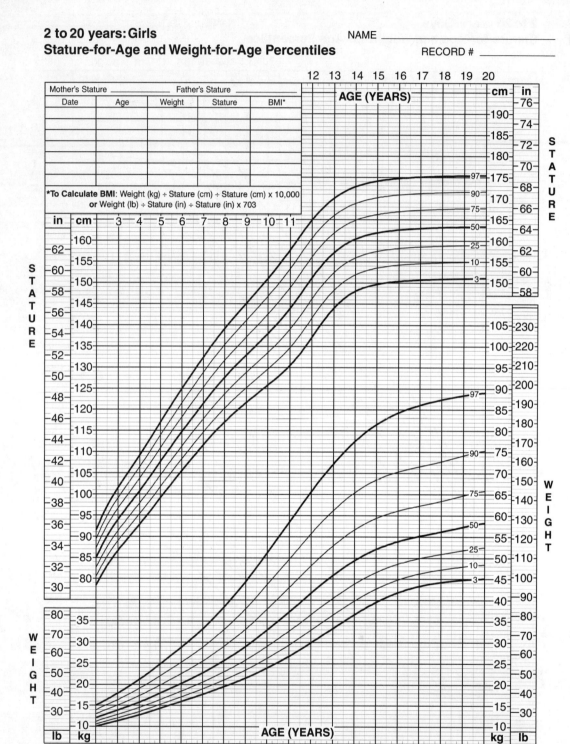

Mother's Stature		Father's Stature		
Date	Age	Weight	Stature	BMI*

*To Calculate BMI: Weight (kg) ÷ Stature (cm) ÷ Stature (cm) x 10,000
or Weight (lb) ÷ Stature (in) ÷ Stature (in) x 703

Source: Developed by the National Center for Health Statistics in collaboration with the National Center for Chronic Disease Prevention and Health Promotion (2000). Online: http://www.cdc.gov/growthcharts.